REABLEMENT IN LONG-TERM CARE FOR OLDER PEOPLE

Transforming Care

Series Editors: **Costanzo Ranci**,
Polytechnic University of Milan and
Tine Rostgaard, Stockholm University
and Roskilde University

Transforming Care provides a crucial platform for scholars researching
early childhood care, care for adults with disabilities and long-term care
for frail older people. The series considers four dimensions of social care:
the institutional setting of care systems and policy; care arrangements
and practices; social and policy innovation for care services and
arrangements and formal and informal care work.

Also available

A Care Crisis in the Nordic Welfare States?
Care Work, Gender Equality and Welfare State Sustainability
Edited by **Lise Lotte Hansen**, **Hanne Marlene Dahl** and **Laura Horn**

Forthcoming in the series:

Unpaid Work in Nursing Homes
Flexible Boundaries
Edited by **Pat Armstrong**

Find out more at
policy.bristoluniversitypress.co.uk/transforming-care

REABLEMENT IN LONG-TERM CARE FOR OLDER PEOPLE

International Perspectives and Future Directions

Edited by
Tine Rostgaard, John Parsons, and Hanne Tuntland

First published in Great Britain in 2024 by

Policy Press, an imprint of
Bristol University Press
University of Bristol
1-9 Old Park Hill
Bristol
BS2 8BB
UK
t: +44 (0)117 374 6645
e: bup-info@bristol.ac.uk

Details of international sales and distribution partners are available at
policy.bristoluniversitypress.co.uk

British Library Cataloguing in Publication Data
A catalogue record for this book is available from the British Library

ISBN 978-1-4473-5991-3 hardcover
ISBN 978-1-4473-5992-0 paperback
ISBN 978-1-4473-5993-7 ePub
ISBN 978-1-4473-5944-4 ePdf

Cover design: Robin Hawes
Front cover image: istock / Stock Illustrations | Circle

Bristol University Press and Policy Press use environmentally responsible
print partners.

Printed in Great Britain by CPI Group (UK) Ltd, Croydon, CR0 4YY

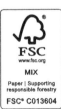

FSC
www.fsc.org
MIX
Paper | Supporting
responsible forestry
FSC® C013604

Contents

List of figures, tables and box   vii

Notes on contributors   ix

PART I   Reablement in contexts, ideas, and implementation

1   Introduction: The concept, rationale, and implications of reablement   3
     Tine Rostgaard, Hanne Tuntland, and John Parsons

2   Perspectives on institutional characteristics, model features,   21
     and theories of reablement
     Hanne Tuntland, John Parsons, and Tine Rostgaard

3   The ideas of reablement and their travel across time and space   46
     Marte Feiring, Oddvar Førland, Fiona Aspinal, and Tine Rostgaard

4   Reablement as an evolution in home care: a comparison of   68
     implementation across five countries
     John Parsons, Elissa Burton, Lea Graff, Silke Metzelthin,
     Hilary O'Connell, and Hanne Tuntland

PART II   Outcomes

5   Does reablement improve client-level outcomes of   93
     participants? An investigation of the current evidence
     Gill Lewin, John Parsons, Hilary O'Connell, and Silke Metzelthin

6   Examining client-level outcomes and instruments in reablement   118
     Hanne Tuntland, Daniel Doh, Maria Ranner, Susanne Guidetti, and
     Magnus Zingmark

7   Reablement as a cost-effective option from a health   137
     economic perspective
     Magnus Zingmark, Hanne Tuntland, and Elissa Burton

PART III   Experience

8   Reablement and dementia   163
     Miia Rahja and Jette Thuesen

9   Better care, better work? Reablement in Danish home care   189
     and the implications for care workers
     Tine Rostgaard and Lea Graff

PART IV   Future perspectives

10   How can we help? Promoting autonomy-compatible help to   219
     reable older adults
     Amy Clotworthy and Rudi Westendorp

11   A cross-country reflection on empirical and theoretical   238
      learnings, challenges, and the way forward for reablement
      John Parsons, Hanne Tuntland, Michelle Nelson, Rudi Westendorp,
      and Tine Rostgaard

Index   248

List of figures, tables and box

Figures

2.1	Overview of the theories underpinning reablement at a grand, meta-range, mid-range, and micro-range level	39
3.1	An illustration of how ideas of active and healthy ageing may have travelled	60
7.1	Development of HRQoL over time in relation to two different interventions	139
7.2	The cost-effectiveness plane for the included studies	153
9.1	Finding work interesting and meaningful, relative to the frequency of providing reablement. Home care workers, per cent	202
9.2	Changes in opportunities for meeting client needs in recent years, relative to the frequency of providing reablement. Home care workers, per cent	203
9.3	Providing individualised care, relative to the frequency of providing reablement. Home care workers, per cent	205
9.4	Have team meeting with middle manager, relative to the frequency of providing reablement. Home care workers, per cent	206
9.5	Support from middle manager, relative to the frequency of providing reablement. Home care workers, per cent	208
9.6	Have lately seriously considered resigning, relative to the frequency of providing reablement. Home care workers, per cent	209

Tables

2.1	Main regional characteristics of the seven countries in the book	22
2.2	Institutional characteristics of the reablement models in the seven countries	24
5.1	Studies examined and summary of their results	96
6.1	Client-level outcomes and measurement instruments in reablement studies	120
6.2	Unique client-level outcomes	126
6.3	Measurement instruments used for client-level outcomes	128
7.1	Identified health economic papers including grey and peer-reviewed literature	144
8.1	Techniques that can be adopted in reablement for individuals with dementia	169
8.2	Reablement intervention programmes for individuals with dementia	171

Box

2.1   Common model features in reablement   32

Notes on contributors

Fiona Aspinal holds a PhD in politics/health sciences and has a background as a nurse. She works as a Senior Research Associate at University College London. Using qualitative and mixed-methods approaches, she has undertaken several complex evaluations of systems, services, and interventions across health and social care settings, including palliative care, community neurological services, support for carers of people with dementia, and reablement. One of her key reablement publications is: Aspinal, F., Glasby, J., Rostgaard, T., Tuntland, H., and Westendorp, R. (2016) 'New horizons: reablement – supporting older people towards independence', *Age and Ageing*, 45(5): 574–8.

Elissa Burton is a Level 2 accredited sports scientist and Senior Research Fellow at the Curtin School of Allied Health and at Curtin enAble Institute, University in Perth, Australia. Burton has explored numerous aspects of physical activity promotion and participation in reablement and home care in general both in Australia initially, and also in Norway through mentoring a Norwegian PhD student. She has conducted numerous research projects with community care organisations in Australia in the areas of falls prevention and physical activity. She currently holds a National Health and Medical Research Council Investigator Grant and is an inaugural (Australian) member of the ReAble Network. Among her reablement publications is: Mjøsund, H.L., Moe, C.F., Burton, E., and Uhrenfeldt, L. (2020) 'Integration of physical activity in reablement for community dwelling older adults: a systematic scoping review', *Journal of Multidisciplinary Healthcare*, 13: 1291–1315.

Amy Clotworthy holds a PhD in ethnology and is Assistant Professor at the University of Copenhagen, Denmark. In her position at the Department of Public Health and the Center for Healthy Aging, her research focuses on how health and social policies targeting older people influence the sociocultural dynamics of later life, and how certain initiatives affect both health professionals and older people in their everyday lives. She coordinates the interdisciplinary research project, 'Standing together – at a distance: how Danes are living with the corona crisis', and she is co-editor of the journal *Anthropology & Aging*. Clotworthy is the author of 'Empowering the elderly? How "Help to Self-help" interventions shape ageing and eldercare in Denmark' (Transcript Verlag, 2021).

Daniel Doh is a social worker and a social policy analyst. Doh is Lecturer at Western Sydney University with an extensive industry experience in aged care and reablement. Daniel Doh's work spans different country contexts including Australia, Ghana, Kenya, Nigeria, and Sierra Leone. He is interested in research on ageing and aged care services for culturally and linguistically diverse communities, quality of life in old age, social isolation and loneliness, social protection, and program evaluation. One of his reablement articles is: Doh, D., Smith, R., and Gevers, P. (2019) 'Reviewing the reablement approach to caring for older people', *Ageing & Society*, 40(6): 1371–83.

Marte Feiring is Professor of Public Health and Rehabilitation, Faculty of Health Science, Oslo Metropolitan University, Norway. She holds a PhD in sociology and a BA in occupational therapy. Her research projects cover historical and critical perspectives on health policies, welfare services, professional knowledge, rehabilitation practices, and civil movements. One of her publications is: Thuesen, J., Feiring, M., Doh, D., and Westendorp, R. (2021) 'Reablement in need of theories of ageing: would theories of successful ageing do?', *Ageing & Society*, 18: 1–13.

Oddvar Førland is Researcher and Professor at the Centre for Care Research, Western Norway University of Applied Sciences, and at the Norwegian University of Science and Technology. He is a sociologist with healthcare and long-term care research as areas of expertise. For several years he has led and participated in projects directed by the Research Council of Norway, ministries, directorates, and municipalities. Førland has published comprehensively about reablement, especially on professional roles and societal perspectives. He is the Chief Editor of the scientific *Journal of Care Research/Tidsskrift for omsorgsforskning*. One of his reablement publications is: Hjelle, K.M., Tuntland, H., Førland, O., and Alvsvåg, H. (2017) 'Driving forces for home-based reablement: a qualitative study of older adults' experiences', *Health & Social Care in the Community*, 25(5): 1581–9.

Lea Graff is Senior Research Analyst at VIVE – The Danish Center for Social Science Research. Her primary research area is community health and social care for older adults. She deals in particular with reablement in home care services and its significance for citizens and healthcare professionals. Currently (2020–23), Lea is engaged in comparative analyses of how home care reablement in Denmark and Norway is influenced by contextual factors as part of her PhD education. Lea is part of several international research collaborations on elder care in the Nordic countries. One key publication is: Rostgaard, T. and Graff, L. (2016) 'Med hænderne i lommen: Borger og medarbeideres samspill og samarbeide i rehabiltering' ('Assisting you with my hands in my pockets – clients' and professionals' interaction and collaboration in reablement') (KORA-report).

Susanne Guidetti is Professor in occupational therapy and has a position at Karolinska Institutet (KI) in Sweden. Her knowledge and experience of planning, developing, and implementing complex interventions as ASSIST using RCT design combined with both qualitative and quantitative methods in Sweden, Denmark, Uganda, and Kenya within healthcare science and rehabilitation. Furthermore, Susanne is a research group leader for the HELD research group at KI. An earlier reablement publication is: Bergström, A., Borell, L., Meijer, S., and Guidetti, S. (2019) 'Evaluation of an intervention addressing a reablement programme for older, community-dwelling persons in Sweden (ASSIST 1.0): a protocol for a feasibility study', *BMJ Open*, 9(7): e025870.

Gill Lewin has recently retired from paid employment but retains Adjunct Professorship at Curtin University in Western Australia. Lewin conducted research on reablement for 16 years when working as Research Director at Silver Chain, where she and colleagues were able to develop and implement the Home Independence Program. Lewin is currently a Board Director of the Australian Association of Gerontology (AAG) and on the Steering Committee of the AAG Research Trust. One of her many reablement publications is: Lewin, G., Concanen, K., and Youens, D. (2016) 'The Home Independence Program with non-health professionals as care managers: an evaluation', *Clinical Interventions in Aging*, 11: 807–17.

Silke Metzelthin is Assistant Professor at Maastricht University in the Netherlands. Her research line focuses on the development and evaluation of innovative care approaches for frail older people. She developed several Dutch reablement (training) programs in co-creation with relevant stakeholders. The feasibility, effectiveness, and cost-effectiveness of these programs were tested by Metzelthin and her colleagues in several pilot studies and three randomised controlled trials. One of her key publications is: Rooijackers, T.H., Kempen, G.I., Zijlstra, G.R., van Rossum, E., Koster, A., Lima Passos, V. and Metzelthin, S. (2021) 'Effectiveness of a reablement training program for homecare staff on older adults' sedentary behavior: a cluster randomized controlled trial', *Journal of the American Geriatrics Society*, 69: 2566–78.

Michelle Nelson holds a PhD in pharmacy. She is a scientist at the Collaboratory for Research and Innovation in Lunenfeld-Tanenbaum Research Institute, Sinai Health System and Assistant Professor in the Institute of Health Policy, Management and Evaluation, University of Toronto, Canada. Michelle is the Chair of the Third Sector Organisations in Integrated Care Special Interest Group with the International Foundation for Integrated Care. A publication of hers is: Nelson, M.L., McKellar, K.A., Yi, J., Kelloway, L., Munce, S., Cott, C., et al (2017) 'Stroke rehabilitation evidence and comorbidity: a systematic scoping review of randomized controlled trials', *Topics in Stroke Rehabilitation*, 24(5): 374–80.

Hilary O'Connell is an occupational therapist and is the Wellness and Reablement Lead at Independent Living Assessment in Western Australia. O'Connell has worked within the reablement field for many years as a clinician and manager of reablement services, allied health, and community care assessment services. She was part of the research, development, and delivery of the first reablement service in Australia – The Home Independence Program, and worked closely with the Western Australian Department of Health to implement reablement focused community care reforms. One of her co-authored studies includes: Burton, E., Lewin, G., O'Connell, H. and Hill, K.D. (2018) 'Falls prevention in community care: 10 years on', *Clinical Intervention in Aging*, 13: 261.

John Parsons is Associate Professor and physiotherapy programme lead at the University of Auckland in New Zealand. He has been central to the design, delivery, and evaluation of reablement type services in New Zealand for 20 years. He was the Associate Editor for *Health & Social Care in the Community* from 2019 to 2022, and has published widely around health services to support older people and those with a disability. His publications include three large randomised controlled trial evaluations of reablement type services in New Zealand. A key recent publication relating to reablement is: Parsons, M., Parsons, J., Pillai, A., Rouse, P., Mathieson, S., Bregmen, R., Smith, C. and Kenealy, T. (2019) 'Post-acute care for older people following injury: a randomized controlled trial', *Journal of the American Medical Directors Association*, 21(3): 404–9.

Miia Rahja is a post-doctoral research associate with Flinders Health and Medical Research Institute, Flinders University, Australia. Her research focuses on evaluating the economic and social impacts of aged and dementia care programs and clinical quality indicators in dementia care. One of her publications is: Clemson, L., Laver, K., Rahja, M., Culph, J., Scanlan, J.N., Day, S., et al (2021) 'Implementing a reablement intervention, "Care of People with dementia in their Environments (COPE)": a hybrid implementation-effectiveness study', *The Gerontologist*, 61(6): 965–76.

Maria Ranner holds a PhD in occupational therapy and has a position as Associate Professor at Luleå University of Technology in Sweden. Her research experience is in reablement and she is a member of the international researcher's network ReAble. Ranner also has research experience in planning and developing complex interventions in the field of rehabilitation. One of her reablement articles is: Ranner, M. and Vik, K. (2020) 'Discourses of service recipients in the context of reablement in Norway', *Scandinavian Journal of Occupational Therapy*: 28(3): 201–12.

Tine Rostgaard is Professor at the Department of Social Sciences and Business at Roskilde University, Denmark, and Professor at the Department of Social Work at Stockholm University, Sweden. She holds a PhD in comparative welfare analysis and specialises in research on care policies and practices in parental leave, childcare, and long-term care. Tine was the initiator of the international researcher network ReAble. She is the co-chair of the international researcher network Transforming Care, http://www.transforming-care.net/ and is presently co-editing the *Handbook of Social Care* for Elgar Publishing. Among her publications related to reablement is: Metzelthin, S., Rostgaard, T., Parsons, M., and Burton, E. (2020) 'Development of an internationally accepted definition of reablement: a Delphi study', *Ageing and Society*, 42(3): 703–18.

Jette Thuesen is Associate Professor at the Unit for User Perspectives and Community Interventions, Department of Public Health, University of Denmark, and at the Center for Rehabilitation and Nutrition, University College Absalon. Her research focuses on ageing and dementia, in particular on the interplay of everyday life practices and institutional arrangements. One of her publications is: Thuesen, J., Feiring, M., Doh, D., and Westendorp, R. (2021) 'Reablement in need of theories of ageing: would theories of successful ageing do?', *Ageing and Society*, 18: 1–13.

Hanne Tuntland is an occupational therapist who holds a position as Professor at Western Norway University of Applied Sciences and a position as an Associate Professor at Oslo Metropolitan University. Her research interests are reablement, rehabilitation, gerontology, and occupational therapy. She has been part of a randomised controlled trial and a nationwide clinical controlled trial on reablement in Norway. As such, Hanne Tuntland is a pioneer in Norwegian reablement research. Moreover, Hanne Tuntland is currently the coordinator of the international researcher's network ReAble. Among her reablement publications is her PhD thesis: 'Reablement in home-dwelling older adults' (University of Bergen, 2017).

Rudi Westendorp is Professor of Medicine at Old Age at the Faculty of Health and Medical Sciences at the University of Copenhagen, Denmark. In this capacity, he performs state-of-the-art and interdisciplinary research within the Department of Public Health and the Center for Healthy Aging. In 2014, he published *Growing Older without Feeling Old*, an international bestseller on vitality and ageing that has been translated into ten languages. Westendorp is the principal investigator of the research consortium, Data for

Good Science – Harnessing the Power of Big Data to Address the Societal Challenge of Aging. One of his reablement publications is: Clotworthy, A., Kusumastuti, S., and Westendorp, R. (2021) 'Reablement through time and space: a scoping review of how the concept of "reablement" for older people has been defined and operationalised', *BMC Geriatrics*, 21(1): 1–16.

Magnus Zingmark is an occupational therapist who has a position as Head of Research and Development at the Health and Social Care Administration in the Municipality of Östersund, as Assistant Researcher at the Department of Health Sciences at Lund University, and is also guest researcher at Umeå University (Sweden). He has led randomised and non-randomised trials, and observational studies in Sweden focused on health promotion, falls prevention, rehabilitation, and reablement. Zingmark is a pioneer in municipality-based research on reablement in Sweden and is currently a member of the steering group of the international researcher's network Reable. The title of his thesis is 'Occupation-focused and occupation-based interventions for community-dwelling older people: intervention effects in relation to facets of occupational engagement and cost effectiveness' (University of Umeå, 2015).

PART I

Reablement in contexts, ideas, and implementation

Introduction: The concept, rationale, and implications of reablement

Tine Rostgaard, Hanne Tuntland, and John Parsons

The aim of the book

With ageing societies, we need to identify sustainable and person-centred solutions for supporting frail older people at home and in ways that improve their quality of life and longevity. There is also a need for innovative and integrative approaches to health and long-term care that are cost-effective and ensure the ageing individual receives individually tailored assistance. Reablement may be an appropriate response to these challenges. It is a radically different approach to home care for older people, seeking to help them to regain and maintain their functional ability and independence, in contrast to more passively providing help and assistance, which has been the traditional approach in compensatory home care (Aspinal et al, 2016; Cochrane et al, 2016). Thus, reablement may be a more sustainable solution for nation-states, municipalities, and service providers to address the needs of an ageing population. Reablement's integrative approach may also help counter the expected increase in public spending on health and long-term care, which is expected to double in the OECD countries by 2060 (de la Maisonneuve and Martins, 2015). However, reablement also implies a new approach to ageing and the provision of social care, which has implications for individuals and their families, as well as for practitioners with regards to new roles, collaborations, needs fulfillment, and obligations. This is why a critical investigation of reablement is needed.

There is already wide and global interest in reablement from policy makers, practitioners, and the academic community. However, since reablement is a relatively new and unexplored approach, research into reablement models and their outcomes has been scarce, uncoordinated, and lacking focus, both nationally and internationally (Legg et al, 2016; Pettersson and Iwarsson, 2017; Clotworthy et al, 2021). In order to bring the research forward and to facilitate theorisation and learning across countries, this book provides an interdisciplinary, comparative, and critical investigation of reablement. Based on collaborations within an international and interdisciplinary research network of reablement researchers, ReAble (https://reable.auckland.ac.nz/), we now take the opportunity to coherently address what reablement is, and what its implications may be on both an individual and societal level.

Our aim with this book is to critically investigate and advance knowledge about reablement in an interdisciplinary and international context: what is the idea behind reablement, which different models exist in different countries, how do they work, and what are the overall consequences for clients and their families, care providers, and societies overall? The research gathered in this book presents empirical evidence on reablement from different Western world countries and with a particular focus on seven countries: Australia,[1] Denmark, England, the Netherlands, New Zealand, Norway, and Sweden, and considers the theoretical implications of the practice. As such, we hope it will be relevant and provide inspiration to academics and practitioners, and that it can be used in the development of international, national, and local policy making.

Why reablement?

Reablement is a response to the need for adapting the health and social care systems to expected changes in the demographic composition of populations in many Western countries. Societies around the world are ageing; in some countries, faster than in others. Population ageing is the fortunate consequence of longer life expectancy but also of declining fertility rates; combined, it means that many countries will have an increasing share of populations aged 65 or over in the years to come. Within less than a century, across OECD countries, older populations aged 65+ will increase on average from less than 9 per cent of the population in 1960 to 27 per cent in 2050. They will make up nearly 40 per cent in countries like Greece, Japan, Portugal, South Korea, and Spain. Population ageing is taking place more rapidly in particular countries and will therefore require more immediate societal adaptions, such as in China where the population aged 65+ will nearly triple between 2015 and 2050, reaching a level just below the OECD average (OECD, 2019).

On average, people around age 65 are well functioning and can manage their daily activities; thus, they are not likely to require any support from health and social care within the subsequent years of their life. However, this is less likely once they reach age 80 and over. There are varied interpretations of the impact of ageing over disability, but some research indicates that there will be an increasing incidence of disability as populations aged 80 and over increase in the OECD countries (Lafortune and Balestat, 2007).

Countries worldwide are therefore facing demographic changes that require societal adaption. An ageing population does not only require an increase in the need for social and healthcare services; it also points to a potential decline in the labour supply, which has implications for the economy. Population ageing will result in fewer taxable incomes, as well as a reduction in workers in the long-term care (LTC) sector, which is already suffering from understaffing and problems with recruitment and retention (OECD, 2020). Therefore, many countries apply a focus on cost-effective approaches that enable redistribution of resources to those who require the most care, often prioritising resources to the degree that LTC needs are unmet and care poverty is created, even in the typically generous Nordic countries (Kröger et al, 2019). As often argued politically as a combined rationale, reablement may instead offer an approach that reduces the need for LTC by actually reducing need for care, as well as enabling a person-centred approach that focuses on what matters to the individual and their quality of life. In other words, reablement has the potential to change the way societies approach LTC policies and implement them into practice.

Reablement can thus be seen as a risk-minimisation strategy that helps older individuals adapt to age-related changes, and may help to prevent certain dependencies. It can also be seen as a policy tool that offers welfare states a new capacity for more dynamically managing and addressing the societal risks associated with population ageing (Rostgaard, 2015). Therefore, one aim of the book is to critically test these rationales and investigate the implications for individuals and societies. The book also seeks to advance the knowledge about reablement in an interdisciplinary and international context.

What is reablement and how is it related to rehabilitation?

Reablement is part of the more inclusive concept of rehabilitation. The World Health Organization defines rehabilitation as 'a set of interventions designed to optimise functioning and reduce disability in individuals with health conditions in interaction with their environment' (World Health Organization, 2017: 1). In this book, we consider 'rehabilitation' to be an umbrella term for many kinds of specific interventions, such as community-based rehabilitation and stroke rehabilitation; reablement is also a rehabilitation intervention under this umbrella.

Ideally, reablement implies the provision of active, person-centred, and goal-oriented support; it should be seen as an alternative to other types of support that merely compensate for care needs and thereby increase the risk of the client becoming passive. The different national – and indeed local – approaches are similar in that reablement is a short-term and intensive intervention that typically lasts 4–6 weeks (Rostgaard, 2015; Tuntland et al, 2015; Legg et al, 2016; Pettersson and Iwarsson, 2017). During this time, an interdisciplinary team composed of social-care workers, nurses, occupational therapists, and physiotherapists cooperate with the older person to identify and work towards a specific outcome goal. The goal is often related to improving functional ability and gaining independence in daily activities, such as shopping, cleaning, or general physical mobility – with an aim to delay or prevent the need for health and social care services – and to increase quality of life (Aspinal et al, 2016; Tuntland et al, 2019). The goal may also be related to social engagement and participation in meaningful social activities. The reablement intervention typically takes place in both the home and local community and is based on training and adaptations in daily activities, physical training, home modifications, and assistive devices. It may also include the involvement of social networks.

Reablement is an active process that involves working alongside the older individual and their family/carers to identify goals for the reablement episode (Parsons et al, 2014). Reablement may also empower the individual and their family/carers within the process (defined as control over one's life, enabling decision-making and self-determination) (Hurst, 2003). In fact, understanding the client's own priorities and concepts of independence is considered to be key to the potential for enhanced effectiveness (Wilde and Glendinning, 2012; Clotworthy, 2020). Also, there is a focus on maximising/optimising function.

Reablement may include a focus on compensatory strategies, defined by the World Health Organization (2012) as adaptive behaviours or alternative ways of performing tasks that enable the individual to optimise their independence despite the impairments and limitations. In many cases, reablement services seek to improve the older individual's social participation (Meyer et al, 2014). Maintaining physical function allows older people to continue in meaningful activities and roles within their communities. Interpreting healthy ageing in this way allows for a refocus from merely the absence of disability to a consideration of wellbeing, participation, and values (Stephens et al, 2015; Stephens and Breheny, 2018).

A common definition of reablement

In order to advance a common understanding and definition of what reablement is across national and disciplinary contexts, the ReAble Network conducted a Delphi study in 2018–19 that aimed to reach agreement on the characteristics, components, goals, and target groups of reablement. The Delphi technique is a widely used consultation process that surveys a panel of experts in order to arrive at a group opinion (Hasson et al, 2000). In this case, our aim was to develop agreement on a generic definition that could simultaneously incorporate the national and indeed local variations in reablement models. In 2020, an internationally accepted definition of reablement was published, based on four web-based rounds of the survey that had been sent to a total of 112 academics and practitioners (Metzelthin et al, 2020). The chapters in this book all relate to the final definition of reablement, which is as follows:

Reablement is a person-centred, holistic approach that aims to enhance an individual's physical and/or other functioning, to increase or maintain their independence in meaningful activities of daily living at their place of residence and to reduce their need for long-term services. Reablement consists of multiple visits and is delivered by a trained and coordinated interdisciplinary team. The approach includes an initial comprehensive assessment followed by regular reassessments and the development of goal-oriented support plans. Reablement supports an individual to achieve their goals, if applicable, through participation in daily activities, home modifications and assistive devices as well as involvement of their social network. Reablement is an inclusive approach irrespective of age, capacity, diagnosis or setting. (Metzelthin et al, 2020: 11)

Chapter 2 by Tuntland et al further investigates these model features of reablement and how they are applied in the seven countries/jurisdictions covered in the book.

Support of new professional and organisational roles, relationships, and power positions

As indicated in the Delphi definition, the application of reablement implies a new perspective. Reablement challenges us not only in our theoretical understanding of what the problem is and how we are going to solve it, but also with what means. It both requires and supports new roles and relationships across clients, their families, and professionals (Rostgaard and Graff, 2016; Clotworthy, 2020). Ideally, with a person-centred and goal-oriented approach, the individual client is expected to engage in identifying and stating their preferences for independent daily living. It is an invitation but also a requirement to continuously reflect on 'what is important to me', in contrast to traditional home care, which is often based on a one-time professional assessment of need followed by fixed times and tasks over the longer term. Another contrast is that the individual works more closely with the professions in a regular conversation to identify how the reablement intervention may support independent living.

Whether the provider is a nurse assistant, a social care worker, an occupational therapist, or a physiotherapist, an important role for the reablement provider is, therefore, to identify the client's potential and motivation for change and to facilitate such change. Often the daily training is provided by a relatively low-skilled support worker. In the book, we apply the term 'reablement care worker' for this function and skill-level. In basing the daily intervention on the interpretation of the older person's capabilities and resources, the reablement care worker may apply more professional independence and autonomy than is the case for regular home care (as elaborated on in Chapter 9 by Rostgaard and Graff). Also, the reablement care worker engages in an ongoing relationship with professional peers as they are expected to participate in and learn from an interdisciplinary collaboration with other professional groups. This implies a new shared power position of the different professions, where, in particular, occupational therapists and physiotherapists seem to have contributed to the professional perspective of maximising independence in daily activities. Yet, reablement seems generally to be adopted and accepted across professional groups. In a qualitative study regarding task-shifting practices in reablement, in this case task-shifting from physiotherapist to auxiliary nurse, two different practices were identified. The first practice, called boundary-making, was found to generate asymmetric power relations that may limit autonomous work and job satisfaction in teams, while the second practice, boundary-blurring, was found to support collaborative practices that endorse holistic approaches and joint learning (Eliassen and Moholt, 2022). Although the boundary-blurring practice seems to be favourable from both a client and a team perspective, asymmetric power relations also exist in many reablement teams.

The support of the older individual's family members is also an important part of a successful outcome in reablement, and informal carers such as partners may influence a successful outcome (Lauritzen et al, 2017). Finally, provider organisations must adapt culturally and change their organisational set-up approach by introducing new overall aims, and by care managers supporting individuals and teams of reablement care workers. When services are procured, special consideration must go into the creation of incentives for non- and for-profit providers for assisting individuals in gaining more independence. Generally, it is cheaper to do things for people than setting time aside to help them do things themselves. Therefore, funders must accept greater provider flexibility where the aim is the outcome and the input may be adjusted along the way according to the individual's abilities and confidence (Francis et al, 2011) (for more information on funding models, see Chapter 2 by Tuntland et al and Chapter 4 by Parsons et al).

The target group

Reablement also poses challenges with regards to who is the target group. The assumption of active participation and involvement of the client raises the question of whether reablement is for everyone, especially if the belief is that a reablement intervention increases quality of life and leads to more independent living, then it is important to not be too restrictive in who is included as a target group. In fact, according to the Delphi definition, reablement is an inclusive approach irrespective of age, capacity, diagnosis, or setting (Metzelthin et al, 2020). Regardless, and presented in more detail in Chapter 2, it has primarily been home-dwelling older adults with physical health conditions and functional limitations who have been offered reablement. As Chapter 8 by Rahja and Thuesen argues, people with dementia are increasingly considered to be a relevant target group also.

However, reablement has been criticised for being a 'one size fits all' intervention (Legg et al, 2016). Indeed, when setting the criteria for inclusion, it is at times recommended that practitioners should not be guided by preconceived notions of who may benefit; rather, they should go beyond such notions and include those who may at first seem to be too frail (Rabiee and Glendinning, 2011). It is reasonable to assume, however, that not all target groups benefit equally from reablement. Some research has found that people who have bone fractures as their main health condition benefit the most with regards to functioning again in daily activities, while having a neurological disease (other than stroke), dizziness/balance problems, and pain/discomfort may lead to poorer outcomes (Tuntland et al, 2017). One explanation for this may be mindset, motivation, and natural healing. Also, a bone fracture occurs as an acute event with a sudden limitation in daily functioning, and where improvements are expected as the fracture heals.

Gender is also an important factor regarding who benefits from reablement, as women seem to benefit more than men. On the other hand, age seems to be a less relevant factor, as adults aged 18–64 tend to benefit as much as adults aged 65+ (Tuntland et al, 2017). In a large cohort study, effects varied among older adults with different levels of care needs. It was found that older adults who have low care needs at baseline, benefit most from reablement when it comes to improvements in ADL (Yu et al, 2022). Hence, although reablement in theory might be offered to everyone, the benefit is not irrespective of diagnosis, capacity or gender. This suggests that some target groups may need more intensive reablement than others to achieve improvements.

Effect of reablement on outcomes

An important question to consider is whether reablement works more overall in improving healthy lives, and has a cost-saving potential compared to traditional home care. Determining the impact of reablement services on outcomes is an imperative need to create sustainable models that meet the needs of the target group for the service and other key stakeholders such as policy makers and funders of health and social care. But before determining whether reablement works, it is necessary to determine by which standard we measure its effect. Common frameworks to evaluate and measure the effect of complex health interventions that support older people (such as reablement) have a number of key domains. These can consider outcomes for the person receiving the service, outcomes for their family, clinical outcomes (such as physical function), and health and social care outcomes, including cost and service usage (Kozma et al, 1993; Porter, 2010).

Chapter 5 by Lewin et al considers the evidence relating to client-level outcomes of older people who received reablement services. These outcomes commonly measure health and wellbeing at an individual level, based on whether they rate their experience positively and value the outcomes achieved. The most common outcomes considered at the client-level in these studies were daily functioning, physical function and quality of life, which is in line with findings in Chapter 6 by Tuntland et al Lewin et al conclude that the overall evidence is still weak regarding showing that individuals have greater improvement in client-level outcomes following reablement than traditional home care. A number of contributing factors are at play: there is the complexity in combining a very personalised intervention with gold-standard randomised controlled trials, as well as the diversity of outcomes measures which have been used in the different studies. Also, as argued in several chapters of the book, reablement is a very context-driven approach with different agendas and variation in actual reablement models across countries. However, in relation to specific outcomes such as performance of daily activities and quality of life or wellbeing, Lewin et al find the overall evidence seems to be promising. Also, there is a reduced service use and user satisfaction generally seems high. Moreover, in a systematic review and qualitative evidence synthesis of older adults' experiences of reablement including 19 studies, reablement was found to improve older adults' health and wellbeing (Mulquiny and Oakman, 2022). So as argued by Lewin et al in their chapter, in the times of ageing populations it seems a good use of public money to apply an approach that reduces the demand for aged care services and does not negatively impact on individuals' health, function, and wellbeing.

There is also developing evidence of reablement being less costly than traditional home care. Chapter 7 by Zingmark et al presents the available evidence relating to the cost-effectiveness of reablement services, and discusses the health economic perspectives of reablement both from a clinical and future research perspective. The authors also point to the need for considering societal costs, such as the cost for healthcare as well as for informal care, and not only the direct cost for the provider. Again, there are few high-quality studies of cost-effectiveness. The authors conclude that health economic perspectives on reablement are limited to studies conducted in Australia, Scandinavia, and the UK. However, when these studies evaluate reablement in relation to usual care, in all studies except one, reablement resulted in lower costs. Reablement is also found to be a cost-effective intervention in a systematic review (Flemming et al, 2021). In other words, there are indications that reablement has the potential to improve lives without straining the public purse − as well as the potential to enable control over one's life and self-determination.

However, it may be discussed whether this focus on ordinary outcomes such as improvement in daily activities and saving money may mislead us. Chapter 10 by Clotworthy and Westendorp provides an alternative view to the measurement of effectiveness of reablement by proposing that a focus on cost-effectiveness, service use, and clinical outcomes results in reablement service models that do not meet the needs of older people, such as the need for social connectedness. Together, the three chapters highlight the need to understand the important outcomes that can be used to measure the impact when planning and designing reablement services.

The wider implications of reablement

Overall, the introduction of reablement must be considered a 'game changer' in the care of older adults, as the aim is to move from compensating for a loss of functional ability to sustained independence in daily activities. There is a direct line from reablement to the influential Indian philosopher and economist Amartya Sen and his moral framework on the need for the development of individual capabilities in order to sustain what he has called our "individual functionings"; what we as humans do and are, and what makes sense to us too (Sen, 2010). The core idea of reablement is therefore that the client participates in determining and deciding which individual functionings are important, and that upholding such functionings ensures a high quality of life. However, the idea of such individual involvement falls short if the functionings conflict with the person's capabilities and resources, or even with the overall aim of and norms for the provision of health and social care, which tend to be focused on physical functioning. For instance, the person's aim may not be to be functionally independent in housework and cleaning, but rather to gain physical mobility in order to participate in social activities. There may therefore be varied assumptions regarding what a 'successful' intervention is, depending on the individual's goals and whether they match the service levels of the provider organisation.

From a critical perspective, the introduction of reablement also suggests that we adopt a new perspective on LTC as the production of outcomes; that is, the able-bodied and functionally independent client. The intersections of active and successful ageing discourses and the neoliberal agenda of activation, responsibilisation, and individualisation imply that, in order to receive care, the individual is expected to aim for change and accept becoming changed (Clotworthy, 2020). The neoliberal rationality of attending to the body as an individual responsibility in this way becomes embodied with the individual (Rudman, 2015). And it may also become embodied in the organisational practice, if individuals who choose not to become 'reabled' are denied regular services. Therefore, any restructuring of LTC services towards reablement must also consider how those who will not or cannot be part of a reablement intervention have their needs met.

Also, reablement services have become widespread in many Western world countries but the evidence of the effectiveness to date lacks a specific consideration of the impact of cultural factors in considering majority populations only. Little of the published research considers the ethnicity of the participants in studies of reablement, but when described, it is clear that the majority of participants are older people of European descent (see for example, Parsons et al, 2018; Parsons et al, 2019). As a result, it is difficult to determine the effect of reablement services among older people from ethnic minorities within a country or in countries outside of Europe, North America, and Australasia.

The development of a more focused and culturally safe practice that aims to reduce issues of health equity should also be considered, particularly as reablement models spread to other countries. Reablement should be more focused on addressing the needs of culturally diverse groups with potentially marked differences in their views towards rehabilitation, reablement, and wider delivery of health and social care services. This is a key issue that points to the importance of considering the cultural context alongside other major contextual factors when designing and implementing reablement-service delivery models. Such an approach may extend beyond having clinical and functional attributes in disease management with a requirement for an alignment in emotional, cultural, and familial understandings (Sheridan et al, 2017; Kuluski et al, 2019).

The spread of reablement and future considerations

Reablement has become increasingly popular in high-income Western countries; a tendency that will most likely continue. Our current knowledge of which countries have implemented reablement derives mainly from research publications from the same countries, but also from personal contact with stakeholders in these countries. Chapter 3 by Feiring et al outlines how the idea of reablement as policy and practice has travelled across regions worldwide. Following instead the academic publications, also gives an indication of the spread from country to country. The first countries to publish peer-reviewed publications on reablement/restorative care were, in chronological order, the United Kingdom in 1999, followed by the United States (2001), Italy (2002), Canada (2005), Australia (2009), Taiwan (2011), New Zealand (2012), and Ireland (2013). Reablement was implemented locally in Sweden around 1997, while Denmark and Norway implemented it locally from 2007 and 2011, respectively (see also Chapter 2). Since the first scientific publication in Norway in 2014, substantial research on reablement has been published. The first scientific publication from

Denmark was from 2016, followed by Sweden in 2017. Other countries that have published research on reablement more recently, from 2017 onwards, are, in chronological order, the Netherlands, South Korea, Japan, Austria, and Finland. However, even if there is an association between a country's scientific publications and implementation of reablement, the relationship is not one-to-one. While some countries like Denmark, New Zealand and the United Kingdom have implemented reablement across more-or-less the whole country, other countries have implemented it in particular geographical regions, home-based care districts or specific settings. Moreover, some countries like Italy, Austria, and South Korea have only one scientific publication and the publication may not reflect actual implementation of reablement in that country. Lastly, there is increasing interest from professional associations, including the Association of Occupational Therapists, in addition to individual OT scholars who, in some countries, have contacted members of the ReAble Network and shown interest in implementing reablement. These countries include Belgium, China, and Iceland. The extent of implementation in these countries is, however, unknown. To conclude, in total, 16 of the 19 aforementioned countries have publications on reablement demonstrating some interest in, or implementation of, the intervention. However, none of these 19 countries are low- or middle-income countries. Furthermore, there are no publications from the countries in the South American and African region.

Finally, some reflections on future considerations regarding application and implementation of reablement. This book highlights a number of issues that need to be addressed in the design, delivery, and evaluation of reablement services. These are relevant for the ongoing refinement and evolution of reablement within countries that have established service-delivery models. However, there is also a need for critical consideration of these issues in regions, jurisdictions, and countries that are planning to introduce reablement. The book chapters provide valuable insights into these considerations, including the need to consider the motivation for implementing reablement. Furthermore, there needs to be an awareness of the need to clearly define the key model features of reablement that will be delivered at a local level, including the composition of the reablement team. Being explicit about the motivation for implementing reablement and describing the key features within a local, regional, or national rollout will allow for more robust comparison across jurisdictions and will also increase the opportunity for successful outcomes for the older people receiving reablement.

A presentation of the book

The motivation for the book has been to apply an interdisciplinary perspective to critically investigate the idea behind reablement, its application, and implementation in different geographical and systemic contexts and, among other things, its implications for cost–effectiveness and for individuals' outcomes and reablement care workers' job quality. We hope that this book will reach a variety of readers and make them interested in how reablement could change LTC systems by providing a more sustainable and person-centred approach for supporting older people to improve their independence in daily functioning.

In line with the interdisciplinary approach in reablement, the authors represent a diversity of disciplines, including economics, ethnology, exercise science, health science, medicine, nursing, occupational therapy, physiotherapy, political science, public health, rehabilitation science, social work, and sociology. The book covers national and cross–country experiences with evidence from reablement in seven countries/jurisdictions across the world and with different LTC systems (Australia, Denmark, England, the Netherlands, New Zealand, Norway, and Sweden).

The book is structured within a number of overarching themes as follows. The following three chapters focus on the theme of *reablement in contexts, ideas, and implementation*:

Chapter 2 by Tuntland et al presents a contextual investigation of the seven countries that are included in the book, including country-specific information on demographics and long-term care systems. The institutional characteristics of reablement in the seven countries are also presented in the chapter, as are more generic reablement model features and the theoretical aspects for reablement.

Chapter 3 by Feiring et al investigates how ideas of reablement have travelled and materialised into similar policies, activities, and institutional practices of reablement within and across different world regions. Data is presented from interviews with key informants and policy documents and online information resources from governing authorities, representing three world regions. The findings illustrate that the travelling of ideas is complex and characterised by circularity rather than linearity. The findings also indicate that transnational ideas of 'successful ageing', 'active and healthy citizens' have travelled to local and national practice, but also from local bottom-up initiatives to the agendas of supranational organisations.

Chapter 4 by Parsons et al explores the related topic of how reablement was implemented across Denmark, the Netherlands, New Zealand, Norway, and Western Australia. Informed by implementation frameworks, the chapter seeks to determine the shared issues for development, refinement, and spread. This allows for consideration of the key features in the composition of reablement across the five countries/regions, together with an illustration of differences in structuring reablement.

In the next part of the book, we focus on the theme of *outcomes* for the individual and in terms of cost-effectiveness.

Chapter 5 by Lewin et al finds that the available evidence for the effect of reablement on the daily functioning of clients remains weak but nevertheless promising in regard to outcomes such as performance of daily activities, quality of life, wellbeing, and user satisfaction. This aligns well with the content of the next chapter through a summary of the evidence relating to what individuals gain from participating in reablement together with a consideration of why the evidence is still limited and how the situation might be improved.

Chapter 6 by Tuntland et al examines the use of outcomes and instruments to measure the impact of services within reablement research. A comparative analysis of the available literature is utilised to consider the evidence with the authors concluding that there is a lack of consistency regarding client-level outcomes and instruments used in reablement research. They suggest that a core set of client-level outcomes related to performance in activities of daily living, physical functioning, and health-related quality of life should be used to enhance comparison across studies.

Chapter 7 by Zingmark et al is based on a literature review of the health-economic perspectives on reablement, and it provides a summary of existing evidence from both a clinical and future-research perspective. The authors conclude that, compared to usual home-care services, reablement is a cost-effective intervention. However, there is a very low number of publications that include health-economic perspectives on reablement; thus, additional studies are urgently needed.

Following this is a part focusing on the *experience* of reablement. Here, we view the experience of reablement for people with dementia and among reablement care workers.

Chapter 8 by Rahja and Thuesen considers reablement in the context of dementia care and reviews research on reablement intervention programs specifically designed for individuals living with dementia. Reablement in dementia care is a relatively new concept and holds promises for this user group and as applied in nursing homes. Intervention programs consist of strategies to address function-related goals, promote activity engagement, consider behavioural and psychological symptoms related to dementia, and include the individual's social networks. However, several barriers to reablement exist, including stigma attached to the disease and limited health professional knowledge regarding dementia.

Chapter 9 by Rostgaard and Graff describes research conducted in Denmark based on qualitative and quantitative data from two local settings in order to unfold reablement care workers' experiences of how reablement has changed their work. The authors conclude that the implementation of reablement in Denmark indicates that reablement changes the understanding of care work in a way that may eventually result in better retention and recruitment of staff in the health and social care sector.

In a final part of the book, we look into *future perspectives* and provide a discussion of where the field is and how it should move forward.

Chapter 10 by Clotworthy and Westendorp challenges the contemporary reablement practice that focuses on improving older people's physical functionality, often at the cost of enhancing their social connectivity. The authors propose a change in perspective and a commitment to move beyond current professional protocols – a change that requires a paradigm shift. Here, professionals should 'help people help themselves' instead of focusing on set functional outcomes and economic benefits. The authors' critical examination of certain fundamental assumptions in reablement aligns well with the need identified in this introductory chapter to consider the theoretical frameworks used in the current design and delivery of reablement services.

Chapter 11 by Parsons et al concludes the book. The chapter is based on a facilitated on-line discussion between five members of the ReAble Network and on the basis of reading the chapters. Their reflections focus on the convergence/divergence of reablement tracks, the challenges and learnings, as well as the implications for theory, practice, and policy making. The chapter summarises the key learnings and messages from the book and illustrates the potential implications for reablement practice and research.

Terminology in the book

The book presents the perspectives and experiences of authors from across disciplines and across countries. As a result, the terminology for central concepts and functions of reablement has not been standardised. The main terms used and their variations are as follows:

- *Client*: An older person to whom reablement services are being delivered. It is common for these older people to also be referred to as a patient or a service user.
- *Home care*: In the book referred to as usual/conventional/traditional home care. Services provided within an older person's place of residence, excluding residential aged care homes. The overarching goal of home care is to provide health and social care support to individuals that will enable them to maintain their independence and the highest quality of life. Home care is often not time-bound or as intensive as reablement.
- *Older person*: A person aged 65 years or over, however, some countries modify this to include groups that are a focus for targeted support (for example Māori in New Zealand are classified as an older adult from age 55). The term is synonymous with elderly/older adult.
- *Reablement care/support workers*: Formally employed health and/or social care workers/home carers whose main function is to motivate and assist

the client in the daily training. They have in many cases received basic training in aged care and/or healthcare, and supplemental training in reablement. They work with other members of the reablement team such as occupational therapists, registered nurses, other health professionals, or social workers.

• *Restorative home care/home support/care*: A term commonly used in Australia, the US, and New Zealand to describe reablement services.

Acknowledgements

We would like to thank the members of the ReAble Network for constructive comments on previous versions of the chapters. We would also like to extend our thanks to student Cecilie Kristine Kolacinski, Roskilde University, for her assistance with formatting the book. The establishment of the ReAble Network was made possible through funding from The Joint Committee for Nordic research councils in the Humanities and Social Sciences (NOS-HS).

Note
[1] At times, referred to as the jurisdiction of Western Australia, as this was where reablement was initiated.

References

Aspinal, F., Glasby, J., Rostgaard, T., Tuntland, H., and Westendorp, R. (2016) 'New horizons: reablement – supporting older people towards independence', *Age and Ageing*, 45(5): 574–8.

Buma, L., Vluggen, S., Zwakhalen, S., Kempen, I.J.M., and Methzelthin, S.F. (2022) 'Effects on clients' daily functioning and common features of reablement interventions: a systematic literature review', *European Journal of Ageing*. DOI: 10.1007/s10433-022-000693-3

Clotworthy, A. (2020) *Empowering the Elderly? How 'Help to Self-help' Interventions Shape Ageing and Eldercare in Denmark*, Bielefeld, Germany: Transcript Verlag.

Clotworthy, A., Kusumastuti, S., and Westendorp, R. (2021) 'Reablement through time and space: a scoping review of how the concept of "reablement" for older people has been defined and operationalised', *BMC Geriatrics*, 21(1): 1–16.

Cochrane, A., McGilloway, S., Furlong, M., Molloy, D., Stevenson, M., and Donnoly, M. (2016) 'Time-limited home-care reablement for maintaining and improving the functional independence of older adults (Review)', *Cochrane Database of Systematic Reviews*, 10, Art. No.:CD101825.

De la Maisonneuve, C. and Martins, J.O. (2015) 'The future of health and long-term care spending', *OECD Journal: Economic Studies*, 2014(1): 61–96.

Eliassen, M. and Moholt, M. (2022) 'Boundary work in task-shifting practices – a qualitative study of reablement teams', *Physiotherapy Theory and Practice*. DOI: 10.1080/09593985.2022.2064380

Flemming, J., Armijo-Olivo, S., Dennett, L., Lapointe, P., Robertson, D., Wang, J., et al (2021) 'Enhanced home care interventions for community residing adults compared with usual care on health and cost-effectiveness outcomes: a systematic review', *American Journal of Physical Medicine & Rehabilitation*, 100(9): 906–17.

Francis, J., Fisher, M., and Rutter D. (2011) 'Reablement: a cost-effective route to better outcomes', Research Briefing 36, Social Care Institute for Excellence.

Hasson, F., Keeney, S., and McKenna, H. (2000) 'Research guidelines for the Delphi survey technique', *Journal of Advanced Nursing*, 32(4): 1008–15.

Hurst, R. (2003) 'The international disability rights movement and the ICF', *Disability & Rehabilitation*, 25(11): 572–6.

Kozma, C.M., Reeder, C., and Schulz, R.M. (1993) 'Economic, clinical, and humanistic outcomes: a planning model for pharmacoeconomic research', *Clinical Therapeutics*, 15(6): 1121–32.

Kröger, T., Puthenparambil, J.M., and Aerschot, L.V. (2019) 'Care poverty: unmet care needs in a Nordic welfare state', *International Journal of Care and Caring*, 3(4): 485–500.

Kuluski, K., Peckham, A., Gill, A., Gagnon, D., Wong-Cornell, C., McKillop, A., Parsons, J., and Sheridan, N. (2019) 'What is important to older people with multimorbidity and their caregivers? Identifying attributes of person centered care from the user perspective', *International Journal of Integrated Care*, 19(2): 1–15.

Lafortune, G. and Balestat, G. (2007) 'Trends in severe disability among elderly people: assessing the evidence in 12 OECD countries and the future implications'. *OECD Health Working Papers*, No. 26, OECD Publishing, Paris.

Langeland, E., Tuntland, H., Folkestad, B., Førland, O., Jacobsen, F., and Kjeken, I. (2019) 'A multicenter investigation of reablement in Norway: a clinical controlled trial', *BMC Geriatrics*, 19(29).

Lauritzen, H.H., Bjerre, M., Graff, L., Rostgaard, T., Casier F., and Fridberg, T. (2017) *Rehabilitering på ældreområdet – Afprøvning af en model for rehabiliteringsforløb I to kommuner, VIVE*. Copenhagen: VIVE [online], Available from: https://www.vive.dk/media/pure/5362/829188

Legg, L., Gladman, J., Drummond, A., and Davidson, A. (2016) 'A systematic review of the evidence on home care reablement services', *Clinical Rehabilitation*, 30(8): 741–9.

Metzelthin, S., Rostgaard, T., Parsons, M., and Burton, E. (2020) 'Development of an internationally accepted definition of reablement: a Delphi study', *Ageing and Society*, 42(3): 703–18.

Meyer, T., Gutenbrunner, C., Kiekens, C., Skempes, D., Melvin, J.L., Schedler, K., Imamura, M., and Stucki, G. (2014) 'ISPRM discussion paper: proposing a conceptual description of health–related rehabilitation services', *Journal of Rehabilitation Medicine*, 46(1): 1–6.

Mulquiny, L. and Oakman, J. (2022) 'Exploring the experience of reablement: a systematic review and qualitative evidence synthesis of older people's and carers' views', *Health & Social Care in the Community*, 30(5): e1471–83.

OECD (2019) *Health at a Glance 2017: OECD Indicators*, OECD Publishing, Paris.

OECD (2020) *Who Cares? Attracting and Retaining Care Workers for the Elderly*, OECD Publishing: Paris.

Parsons, J., Jacobs, S., and Parsons, M. (2014) 'The use of goals as a focus for services for community dwelling older people', in R.J. Siegert and W. Levack (ed) *Handbook of Rehabilitation Goal Setting*, San Francisco: CRC Press/Taylor & Francis, pp 305–324.

Parsons, M., Parsons, J., Rouse, P., Pillai, A., Mathieson, S., Parsons, R., Smith, C., and Kenealy, T. (2018) 'Supported Discharge Teams for older people in hospital acute care: a randomised controlled trial', *Age & Ageing*, 47(2): 288–94.

Parsons, M., Parsons, J., Pillai, A., Rouse, P., Mathieson, S., Bregmen, R., Smith, C., and Kenealy, T. (2019) 'Post-acute care for older people following injury: a randomized controlled trial', *Journal of the American Medical Directors Association*, 21(3): 404–9.

Pettersson, C. and Iwarsson, S. (2017) 'Evidence-based interventions involving occupational therapists are needed in re-ablement for older community-living people: a systematic review', *British Journal of Occupational Therapy*, 80(5): 273–85.

Porter, M.E. (2010) 'What is value in health care', *New England Journal of Medicine*, 363(26): 2477–81.

Rabiee, P. and Glendinning, C. (2011) 'Organisation and delivery of home care re-ablement: what makes a difference?', *Health & Social Care in the Community*, 19(5): 495–503.

ReAble Network (nd) 'Reablement: restorative home support, a new approach' [online], Available from: https://reable.auckland.ac.nz/

Rostgaard, T. (2015) 'Failing ageing? Risk management in the active ageing society', in M. Frederiksen, J.E. Larsen, and T. Bengtsson (eds) in *Risk and the Modern Welfare State – Sociological Investigations of the Danish Case*, London: Palgrave Macmillan, pp 153–68.

Rostgaard, T. and Graff, L. (2016) *Med hænderne i lommen – Borger og medarbejders samspil og samarbejde i rehabilitering*, VIVE report. Copenhagen: VIVE [online], Available from: https://www.vive.dk/da/udgivelser/med-haenderne-i-lommen-8841/

Rudman, D.L. (2015) 'Embodying positive aging and neoliberal rationality: talking about the aging body within narratives of retirement', *Journal of Aging Studies*, 34: 10–20.

Sen, A. (2010) 'Equality of what?', in S.M. McMurrin (ed) *The Tanner Lectures on Human Values*, 4, Cambridge: Cambridge University Press, pp 195–220.

Sheridan, N., Kenealy, T., Stewart, L., Lampshire, D., Robust, T.T., Parsons, J., McKillop, A., Couturier, Y., Denis, J.-L., and Connolly, M. (2017) 'When equity is central to research: implications for researchers and consumers in the research team', *International Journal of Integrated Care*, 17(2): 14.

Stephens, C. and Breheny, M. (2018) *Healthy Ageing: A Capability Approach to Inclusive Policy and Practice*, London: Routledge.

Stephens, C., Breheny, M., and Mansvelt, J. (2015) 'Healthy ageing from the perspective of older people: a capability approach to resilience', *Psychology & Health*, 30(6): 715–31.

Tuntland, H., Aaslund, M., Espehaug, B., Førland, O., and Kjeken, I. (2015) 'Reablement in community-dwelling older adults: a randomised controlled trial', *BMC Geriatrics*, 15(146): 1–11.

Tuntland, H., Kjeken, I., Folkestad, B., Førland, O., and Langeland, E. (2019) 'Everyday occupations that older adults participating in reablement prioritise: A cross-sectional study', *Scandinavian Journal of Occupational Therapy*: 1–11. DOI: 10.1080/11038128.2019.1604800

Tuntland, H., Kjeken, I., Langeland, E., Folkestad, B., Espehaug, B., Førland, O., and Aaslund, M. (2017) 'Predictors of outcomes following reablement in community-dwelling older adults', *Clinical Intervention in Aging*, 12: 55–63.

Wade, D.T., Smeets, R.J., and Verbunt, J.A. (2010) 'Research in rehabilitation medicine: methodological challenges', *Journal of Clinical Epidemiology*, 63(7): 699–704.

Wilde, A. and Glendinning, C. (2012) '"If they're helping me then how can I be independent?" The perceptions and experience of users of home-care re-ablement services', *Health & Social Care in the Community*, 20(6): 583–90.

World Health Organization (2012) *Guidelines on Health-Related Rehabilitation (Rehabilitation Guidelines)*, Geneva: World Health Organization.

World Health Organization (2015) *WHO Global Strategy on People-Centred and Integrated Health Services: Interim Report*, Geneva: World Health Organization [online], Available from: https://apps.who.int/iris/handle/10665/155002

World Health Organization (2017) *Rehabilitation in Health Systems*, Geneva: World Health Organization. Licence: CC BY-NC-SA 3.0 IGO.

Yu, H.W., Wu, S.C., Chen, H.H., Yeh, Y.P., and Chen, Y.M. (2022) 'Relationships between reablement-embedded home-and community-based service use patterns and functional improvement among older adults in Taiwan', *Health & Social Care in the Community*, 1–11.

Perspectives on institutional characteristics, model features, and theories of reablement

Hanne Tuntland, John Parsons, and Tine Rostgaard

Introduction

As presented in Chapter 1, the Delphi-based definition of reablement is based on the understanding that characteristics, components, goals and target groups are common across national and disciplinary contexts. This chapter builds on the presentation on reablement in Chapter 1, but expands the scope to country-specific demographic information and welfare regimes. It has a comparative perspective presenting main regional characteristics of the countries represented in the book. The intention is that providing this overview will help the reader understand the country-specific contexts when reading the following chapters of the book. More generic reablement model features and theoretical aspects for reablement, are also given broad attention in the chapter.

A contextual presentation of the countries

Table 2.1 presents a cross-country analysis of seven countries: Australia, Denmark, England,[1] the Netherlands, New Zealand, Norway, and Sweden. These countries are included in the book as they are among the ones where reablement as a policy and professional approach is most developed and has the longest history. The countries are situated geographically in four different regions of the world: Australasia (Australia and New Zealand), Scandinavia (Denmark, Norway and Sweden), and western (England) and central Europe (the Netherlands). As investigated in Chapter 3 by Feiring et al, there is a clear pattern of how reablement has travelled across and between countries in these regions, and quite interestingly, the travel between regions is irrespective of their different regional history of welfare regimes and social rights for long-term care. That is, reablement seems to be applied across variations of welfare systems.

Table 2.1: Main regional characteristics of the seven countries in the book

Groups of countries in four geographical regions	Western Europe: United Kingdom	Australasia: Australia and New Zealand	Scandinavia: Denmark, Norway and Sweden	Central-Europe: The Netherlands
Welfare model	Liberal	Liberal	Social democratic	Mixed
Population 65+ as % total population (2019)[1]	UK: 18.5	AU: 15.9 NZ: 16.0	DK: 20.0 SE: 20.2 NO: 17.3	19.6
% GDP for LTC (2019)[1]	UK: 2.3	AU: 1.5 NZ: 1.5	DK: 3.6 N: 3.7 S: 3.4	4.1
Population 65+ with home care (2019)[2]	UK: no data	AU: 8.2 NZ: 8.5	DK: 11.1 N:11.0 S: 11.9	7.7
Population 65+ living in institutional care (2019)[3]	UK: 3.2 (2011)	AU: 5.9 NZ: 4.3	DK: 3.5 SE: 4.2 NO: 4.1	4.2
Life expectancy at birth (2020 or latest year)[4]	UK: 80.4	AU: 83.0 NZ: 82.1	DK: 81.6 N: 83.3 S: 82.5	81.5
Healthy life expectancy at age 60 (2019)[5]	UK: 18.3	AU: 19.0 NZ: 20.8	DK: 18.2 N: 18.5 SE: 18.9	18.4

Notes: [1] OECD (nda); [2] UN (2019); [3] OECD (ndc), NL: 2018. UK: No data for home care. Data on institutional care for UK from 2011 and from ONS (nd); [4] OECD (ndb); [5] World Health Organization (nd); GDP = gross domestic product

Welfare regimes

Table 2.1 presents the three categories of welfare regimes which the countries represent. Australia, United Kingdom (England), and New Zealand represent liberal welfare regimes with low proportions of GDP devoted to long-term care (LTC) (1.5–2.3 per cent; OECD average 1.5 per cent). This welfare regime is also characterised by having minimum but universal public LTC services; instead individualised and market-based care solutions are encouraged. In contrast, in the social-democratic welfare regime, there is universal and affordable provision of relatively generous public LTC services, and a considerable proportion of GDP goes to LTC (between 3.4–3.7 per cent). This is evident in the proportion of persons aged 65+ with home care services (between 11.1–11.9 per cent), which is higher in Scandinavia than in the other countries, also reflecting the policy of de-institutionalisation applied there. The Netherlands represents a mixed model with high GDP investments for LTC (4.1 percent), the highest in fact among OECD countries, but with lower service coverage than in the social-democratic regime, and with emphasis on the role of the family as well as the market (Ranci and Rostgaard, forthcoming).

Ageing and healthy ageing

As presented in Table 2.1, these are also countries where the proportion of older people today constitute a substantial amount of the population, although with a higher share in some countries than in others. Thus, Sweden is the 'oldest' country in the group, with 20.2 per cent of the population being 65 years or older, and Australia the 'youngest' with 15.9 per cent. In comparison, the OECD average is nine per cent (OECD, 2019). Reflecting the relatively high living standards and well-developed health systems in these countries, they all have high life expectancy at birth, between 80–83 years. As many other western countries, they also have ageing populations which live their last years with multiple illnesses. As presented in Table 2.1, the number of remaining years of life with good health at the age of 60 therefore does not match the full remaining lifetime – varying from 18–21 years. In summary, these are ageing societies with more than 15 per cent of the population aged 65+ and average life expectancies well over 80 years, of which some years can be expected to be with functional limitations and disabilities. Therefore, across the countries there is an urgent need for identifying long-term care solutions which are cost-effective and meet the needs of an ageing population.

Reablement models in the seven countries and their institutional characteristics

The influence of ageing populations and financial pressures together with a dominant paradigm of active and successful ageing, has paved the way for reablement in all the countries. Table 2.2. presents a number of the main characteristics of the reablement models in the seven countries in the book. As shown in the table (and further investigated in Chapter 3 by Feiring et al), the *year* of introducing reablement spans over nearly 30 years, the earliest in Sweden (1997) and the latest (locally) in the Netherlands (2015).

The various *terms* applied nationally/locally for reablement are different. As the countries represent different language groups, this could be expected. But the various terms also differ regarding their meaning. The use of various terms (and meanings) does not seem to indicate a policy learning taking place from country to country that reflects the chronological order of when reablement was introduced. As an example, being the second country to introduce reablement, Australia initially referred to 'wellness' and later 'restorative care', instead of the similar term 'everyday rehabilitation' used

Table 2.2: Institutional characteristics of the reablement models in the seven countries

	Australia	Denmark	England[1]	The Netherlands	New Zealand	Norway	Sweden
Year of introducing reablement	Western Australia and Victoria from 1999; nationally from 2018	2007 (locally; nationally and by law 2015)	2000s	2015 (local training program)	From 2000 onwards	From 2011 onwards	1997 (locally; spreading to other municipalities from 2000 onwards)
Term	Originally wellness; today restorative home care/ reablement	(Hverdags) rehabilitering [[Everyday] reablement]	Reablement and intermediate care	Local training programs, for instance Blijf Actief Thuis [Stay Active at Home], but today spreading to country level under various names reflecting enabling ageing in place	Restorative home support	Hverdagsrehabilitering [Everyday reablement]	Vardagsrehabilitering [Everyday reablement]
Overall policy goal	Independence and autonomy	Independence and autonomy, quality of life, cost-saving	Independence, discharge planning, health benefits, preventing and delaying needs for care and support, recovering skills and confidence	Independence and autonomy, wellbeing, ageing-in-place, cost-savings	Wellness, sustainable, culturally appropriate	Independence, activation, mastering, prevention, quality of life	Person-centred care, prevention and maintenance, functional independence, activation
Top-down/ bottom-up policy approach	Bottom-up first; then top-down	Bottom-up first; then top-down	Bottom-up first; then top-down	Bottom-up first; then top-down	Initial work was from small pilot projects but quickly became top-down	Bottom-up	Bottom-up

Table 2.2: Institutional characteristics of the reablement models in the seven countries (continued)

	Australia	Denmark	England[1]	The Netherlands	New Zealand	Norway	Sweden
National investment in evidence	Initially RCT study in Western Australia (Silver Chain)	Development of evidence-based model and pre-/post-evaluation of the model in two municipalities	RCT study financed by Department of Health	National funding for investigation of several pilots and an RCT of the local training program	Funding from central government to determine effectiveness	National funding of CCT research	No
Target group	Older adults 65+ (aboriginal and Torres Strait Islander people 50+) with need for assistance to continue living in the community	Primarily older adults 65+ with functional limitation living in the community		Mainly aimed at 65+	Older adults 65+ (Māori aged over 55 years)	Primarily older adults 65+ with a functional decline living in the community and irrespective of diagnosis	For all age groups
Overall funding model	Tax-financed and means-tested user fees	Tax-financed; no user fees	Tax-financed; means-tested user fees can be applied after the first 6 weeks	Tax-financed; no user fees although not all costs may be covered	Tax-financed; no user fees	Tax-financed; user fees	Tax-financed; no user fees

(continued)

Table 2.2: Institutional characteristics of the reablement models in the seven countries (continued)

	Australia	Denmark	England[1]	The Netherlands	New Zealand	Norway	Sweden
Funding of provider	Fee-per-hour per type of service	Varies between municipalities. Fee-per-hour per type of service, lumpsum	Varies between local councils; can be a block contract, a fee-per-hour contract or an outcomes-based contract	Fee-per-hour or lumpsum funding	Case-mix (funding based on variation of cost according to a validated system of aggregation of patients into groups based on defined characteristics)	Fee-for-service basis with separate compensation on a service level for both physiotherapy and general practitioner input	Varies between municipalities
National guidance and/or coordination of implementation	National guidance and coordination, integration into national home support program, including program manuals	National guidance in two white books on reablement by National Health Board	National guidance	No national guidance or coordination	Integration into national home and community support service specifications	National guidance of implementation of reablement supported in several white books	No national guidance or coordination

Reablement – main perspectives

Table 2.2: Institutional characteristics of the reablement models in the seven countries (continued)

	Australia	Denmark	England[1]	The Netherlands	New Zealand	Norway	Sweden
Take up of reablement, local municipalities/ regions	All home support providers funded under the national home support program are to use a wellness and reablement approach	100% since 2015 but approx. 98% had voluntarily implemented reablement before 2015	Almost all local councils	Local healthcare organisations/ municipalities	National spread across health regions	Three in four municipalities	Not evaluated but most likely all municipalities to some extent, as an intersection with home health services
Assessment	Public. Purchaser/ provider split	Public. Purchaser/ provider split	Depends on the model of provision in each area	Public healthcare provider	Public. Purchaser/ provider split	Public. Purchaser/ provider split	Public. Purchaser/ provider split
Providers (public, for-profit, mix)	A mix of not-for-profit, government and private. However, 2/3 are not for profit	Mix, but mainly public (generally around 1/3 of home help users use a for-profit provider)	Mostly providers are contracted private, for-profit or not-for-profit	Mainly non-profit	All providers are contracted organisations	Providers are publicly funded	Mix, but mainly public

(continued)

Table 2.2: Institutional characteristics of the reablement models in the seven countries (continued)

	Australia	Denmark	England[1]	The Netherlands	New Zealand	Norway	Sweden
Professions involved	Predominantly trained home support workers and coordinators (nursing/OT/PT background)	Health and social care workers (approx. 80% have formal qualifications) and PT/OTs; other professions as needed, such as nurses	Predominantly support workers with some (access to) OT, rarely PT or nurse	Therapists, usually the OT/PT are in charge of the daily training, coordination by OTs	Mainly nurses, unregulated support workers with some PT and OT input as required	PTs, OTs, nurses, auxiliary nurses and unskilled nurse assistants are the core team. Some municipalities have additional professions like social educator	Core team consist of OTs, PTs, nurses, support workers, social care workers Can be called upon: primary care staff
Reablement training	Nationally funded on-line reablement training available to home care providers. Support workers usually require min. training in aged care	Part of curriculum in health and social care worker educations; local training courses, some nationally funded	Provider organisations are responsible for training their staff	Training at organisations' own expenses	Nationally funding for local training courses	Local and regional training courses	Local training courses

Table 2.2: Institutional characteristics of the reablement models in the seven countries (continued)

	Australia	Denmark	England[1]	The Netherlands	New Zealand	Norway	Sweden
Reablement services	Personal care, practical assistance with shopping, laundry, housework shopping, accessing the community and social connections	Personal care, nursing, mobility training, and practical assistance such as house cleaning, meals and laundry. Social support increasingly a task for voluntary agencies	Most services provide personal care, domestic skills, safety, information, getting around inside and outside or home, social activities	All daily activities related to living at home	Personal care, practical assistance, nursing services, social relations/ participation	Includes all daily activities based on what is important for the client	Varies between municipalities. Mainly focused on personal care and indoor mobility

Note: [1] England is used to exemplify the United Kingdom, as there is most information from this country; CCT = clinical controlled trial; CHSP = Commonwealth Home Support Programme; RCT = randomised controlled trial.

by Sweden. Rather, the use of terminology seems to reflect a simultaneous development within regions where countries have to various degrees been inspired by one another (see also Chapter 3 by Feiring et al). Therefore, the term *everyday rehabilitation* is commonly used in Scandinavia, *restorative care* is used in the Australasian region, while *reablement* is used in England (as well as Northern Ireland, Scotland, and Wales) – and reablement is also the term commonly used in the international literature today. In the Netherlands, reablement was in the beginning mainly applied as a local training program with a name that clearly reflects its purpose, '*stay active at home*'. During the last years, reablement programmes have spread slowly but continuously to other parts of the Netherlands. There is no common word for reablement in Dutch and the local provider organisations often decide on a project name that reflects enabling ageing in place, such as 'langer actief thuis' (longer active at home), and 'langer vitaal thuis' (longer vital at home).

As Table 2.2 indicates, across the countries, there is similarity in the *policy/program goals* as these emphasise restoring or maintaining autonomy and independence in everyday activities, as a way to improve quality of life and wellbeing, ensure delay in needs for LTC, and create more financially sustainable LTC systems. In Sweden, there is no overall national policy but the original local program in Östersund municipality emphasised person-centred care by placing the user at the centre. In England also, the possibility of improving discharge procedures is mentioned as a policy goal. Reablement is mainly for older people 65+, but in the Netherlands and Sweden, it is intended for all age groups. In cases of sub-populations considered in risk, the 65+ age limit may be lowered. This is the case in Australia for the aboriginal and Torres Strait islander people, and in New Zealand for the Māori population.

Apart from New Zealand, reablement was in all other places initially started and consolidated as *local bottom-up initiatives* (Table 2.2). In most cases, it spread to all other localities or providers, the exception being Norway, where three in four municipalities offer reablement, and in the Netherlands, where reablement has spread from a local training program to other local areas as policy makers increasingly become interested in the model. Apart from Sweden, there has been national funding allocated for determining the outcome of the reablement intervention. Generally, therefore, it seems that the implementation of reablement is *evidence-based*. Many of the countries provide national *guidance* but no coordination on how to implement reablement, and typically guidance will be found in White papers, but reablement is part of *national legislation* only in Australia (since 2018) and Denmark (since 2015). Only in Denmark are there statistics on the proportion of older people receiving reablement, 3.6 per cent of 65+ in 2018.

As shown in Table 2.2, the overall *funding model* of reablement is based on general taxation in all seven countries, in Australia, England, and Norway supplemented by means-tested user fees – and in England user fees can be applied after the initial first 6 weeks, although this rarely happens. *Funding of providers* vary and only in England it may be result based. Here, some local councils will use outcomes-based commissioning to pay for all services, including reablement. In the case of the other countries, funding is set up as either a fee-per-hour type of service, or lumpsum funding. In New Zealand and the Netherlands respectively, there has been an emphasis on modifying the model of funding to incentivise providers to apply the principles of the model (Parsons et al, 2018; Elissen et al, 2020). In New Zealand, a case-mix funding model was developed and implemented that uses the inter-RAI contact (older people with non-complex needs) and home care assessments (for complex needs) (Parsons et al, 2018).

Assessment of need and appropriateness of reablement is typically performed by a public agency as part of a purchaser-provider split. In England, however, this depends on the model of provision in the area. *Providers* are a mix, and tend, for instance, in Scandinavia to be public, supplemented by for-profit providers, while in England, they are a mix of for-profit and non-profit organisations. In all countries, reablement is based on the *interdisciplinary collaboration* of different professions, organised in teams. In most places (Australia, Denmark and England, and Norway), the person in charge of daily interventions will be a reablement care/support worker, who works closely together with an occupational therapist or physiotherapist to plan and adjust the intervention according to changes in needs. The reablement care/ support workers have in many cases received basic training in aged care and/ or healthcare. In Norway and the Netherlands, the occupational therapist and physiotherapist have a more prominent role in the daily intervention and in New Zealand and the Netherlands the nurse has the central role. Only in Denmark, *training* in reablement is part of general education for reablement care workers, while in most other countries, training is funded nationally and offered locally. In the Netherlands and England, reablement training is based on the organisations funding and offering training.

The *services* delivered by the reablement team will in most cases include training in daily activities related to living at home (Table 2.2). This includes personal care and practical domestic chores, such as cleaning, laundry, and meals. In Sweden, activities are mainly focused on personal care and indoor mobility. In Australia, England, New Zealand, and Norway, activities may include accessing the community and social connection as a means to gain independence, while in Denmark such activities are increasingly turned over to non-profit organisations.

Reablement model features

As illustrated by the aforementioned presentation of the institutional characteristics of the national/local reablement models, there is some commonality in the institutional approach to reablement across the seven countries. This is not to say that there is no variation in the actual implementation of reablement across national and local reablement models, in fact this variation can be considerable – and not all reablement models may comply with the Delphi definition (see Chapter 1 Rostgaard et al for the Delphi definition). Chapter 4 by Parsons et al investigates how some of these variations in implementation are determined. Nevertheless, the seven countries generally apply what can be considered the main model features which are unique to the reablement approach, see Box 2.1, and highlighted in the Delphi definition.

The empirical application of these model features is presented in detail in the following, in order to give a more thorough understanding of what characterises reablement, and how it is different from more traditional approaches to home care. The presentation will draw on various national and comparative studies of reablement and will therefore provide a more general account of reablement models than the previous section on the seven countries.

Box 2.1: Common model features in reablement

- Person-centred intervention
- Targeted at home-dwelling older adults
- In a familiar setting
- Goal-setting and goal-setting instruments
- Holistic approach to goals
- Multimodal intervention components
- An intensive and relation-based intervention
- An interdisciplinary approach
- Regular assessments
- Staff training

Person-centred intervention

According to the Delphi definition, reablement is a person-centred intervention (Metzelthin et al, 2020), and several authors highlight the importance of reablement being a person-centred intervention (Newton, 2012; Aspinal et al, 2016; Tuntland et al, 2019; Azim et al, 2022). The core idea of a person-centred approach to long-term care for older people is to organise services in accordance with what is important to the individual person and centred around the individual (World Health Organization, 2015). In person-centred practice, the question raised to the client is: "What is important to you?". The practice is supported by values of respect for persons, individual right to self-determination, as well as mutual respect and understanding (McGormack et al, 2017: 20).

Targeted at home-dwelling older adults

Although the Delphi definition argues that reablement is an inclusive approach irrespective of age, capacity, diagnosis, or setting (Metzelthin et al, 2020), it has primarily been home-dwelling older adults with somatic health conditions who have been offered reablement (Langeland et al, 2019). In a systematic review of 20 studies involving reablement services, with a total of 6,798 participants, most participants were female: 69.8 per cent (range 21.6–87.5) and had a mean age of 79.5 years old (range 34.5–87.7). Moreover, all interventions were aimed at clients that required assistance with more than one ADL task or experienced functional decline (Buma et al, 2022). Previously, older adults with dementia were excluded from reablement but, to an increasing degree, people with dementia are now considered to be a relevant target group (see Chapter 8 by Rahja and Thuesen for examples and more details on this issue).

In a familiar setting

Reablement takes place in the client's 'place of residence' according to the international definition (Metzelthin et al, 2020: 11). The fact that reablement takes place in a familiar setting is a valuable feature of the intervention that is not often recognised in the literature but is nonetheless assumed to be an important success factor. Hence, "being at home with my stuff and my people" is found to be an important factor (Hjelle et al, 2016: 5). When individuals are engaged in 'real' task performance, in 'real' places, with 'real' objects with the 'real' people present, then they 'really' do it and the task performance is fully contextualised (Fisher and Marterella, 2019). This is the case in reablement: A man who wants to improve his skills in preparing a meal would do so at home under the guidance of a reablement care/support worker; in his own kitchen, equipped with his own kitchen utensils that he usually uses, he would prepare a dish that he wants to be able to prepare, primarily at a time when he would usually prepare it. This is in contrast to hospital-based rehabilitation which has fewer situational elements, making the rehabilitation process less contextualised and authentic.

Goal-setting and goal-setting instruments

In reablement, it is essential that the individual defines their own goals in collaboration with the reablement providers. Goal-setting allows individuals to identify and prioritise daily activities that they find difficult to perform and important to improve or, as it is phrased in the Norwegian reablement approach, to identify 'what activities are important in your life now?' Focusing on the individual's goals also functions as a unifying platform in the interprofessional team (Birkeland et al, 2017). Older adults identify goals as an important motivator and attainment of goals have a positive impact on their reablement experience (Mulquiny and Oakman, 2022). In a recent scoping review including 21 studies, goal-setting was found to be the most frequently used behaviour change technique in reablement (Azim et al, 2022), illustrating the understanding that the goal-setting process potentially can lead to positive behaviour change. This is because intentions or goals set the stage for behaviour change. Goals may enable clients to return to what matters most to them (Azim et al, 2022). As a result, goal-setting promotes motivation, which may be a key to success in reablement (Tuntland et al, 2017). It is common to use an assessment method or specific instruments to identify activities that the client finds meaningful and to develop a person-centred and goal-oriented support plan (Buma et al, 2022). In several countries, the person-specific instrument Canadian Occupational Performance Measure (COPM) is being used (Law et al, 2015), but the use of instruments varies across national settings. As an example, in New Zealand, the instrument Towards Achieving Realistic Goals for Elders Tool (TARGET) is used (Parsons and Parsons, 2012). It is worth noting that use of a standardised goal-setting instrument, may lead to more positive outcomes regarding daily functioning (Buma et al, 2022).

Holistic approach to goals

Being a holistic intervention means in this respect taking into account various aspects of the client's health and functioning, and to incorporate these aspects in the client's goals. To increase or maintain an individual's independence in meaningful daily activities is often considered to be the most essential goal in reablement. However, the understanding of goals must go beyond the dependence/independence continuum, since advances in ADL may be due to changes in self-efficacy and feelings of improved safety and confidence, and not only improvement in physical functioning. In other words, physical functioning is a means to maintain everyday life (Bergström et al, 2022). Hence, goals frequently relate to self-care and physical functioning, for instance to be able to dress oneself, or to be able walk to the nearby grocery store. Still, goals may also be leisure activities and of psychosocial character, such as doing handicrafts or be able to visit friends and family, as documented by Tuntland et al in a large cross-sectional study identifying clients' goals in reablement (2019). This is however contested, as it is argued that having a social life is rarely included in the goals of reablement programs

(Mulquiny and Oakman, 2022). Likewise, Clotworthy and Westendorp argue in Chapter 10 that reablement focuses on improving older people's physical functionality, often at the cost of taking care of social needs. It is worth noticing that a person–centred approach in the goal-setting process is a prerequisite for enhancing social goals to be set. Nonetheless, in order for reablement to fully be a holistic intervention, more attention should be given to the social needs of the clients.

Multimodal intervention components

Reablement is a multimodal intervention with application of several components. The most common interventions components to reach clients goals are in a systematic review including 20 studies found in declining order to be ADL-training, physical and/or functional exercise, education and environmental adaptations (Buma et al, 2022). *ADL-training* was an intervention component included in all studies in the review, of which the review also found promising results, and includes individual training in everyday activities such as personal care and domestic chores. The client is learning by doing while the reablement provider simplifies, adapts, and gradually increases the demands entailed in the activity. *Physical and/or functional exercises* focus on physical activity by means of training muscle strength, balance, endurance, and fine motor skills. Training can both be provided individually and in group sessions. *Education* plays a role in reaching client's goals. Clients are taught self-management, building confidence, healthy ageing, problem-solving and medication use. Finally, *environmental adaptations* imply use of assistive technology and home modifications. An intervention component found in the review to be more seldom used was *functional disorder management*, such as management of pain, continence, nutrition, skin integrity, testing of blood and urine, and management of medication. The review concludes that it seems like effective interventions on average include more diverse components and that the effective interventions include on average four components (Buma et al, 2022).

An intensive and relation-based intervention

Generally, reablement is an intensive intervention, based on efforts provided by the professionals in the reablement team. The degree of intensity is based on the frequency of home visits and individual training, as well as the duration of the intervention. In a large study that found that reablement had an effect on the performance of daily activities, physical function, and quality of life, reablement was offered on average daily for 5.7 weeks (Langeland et al, 2019). If the approach is diluted with weaker intensity, it is uncertain whether the intervention would still have an effect. This may be part of the reason why no effect was found in a randomised controlled trial in which reablement was offered only once a week for 6 weeks (Chiu et al, 2021). In a systematic review, reablement had a mean duration of 15.7 weeks. The effective interventions had slightly shorter duration compared to the non-effective interventions (Buma et al, 2022). In addition, as pointed out by Rostgaard and Graff in Chapter 9, the frequency of home visits and the close relational contact with the individual is found to be associated with care workers having more meaningful work and professional autonomy.

An interdisciplinary approach

Reablement is per definition an interdisciplinary intervention, often involving collaboration across social and health professions. However, the actual skills mix of professions involved in reablement varies between countries and localities. In the systematic review of Buma et al most interdisciplinary teams consisted of registered nurses, nursing assistants, occupational therapists and physiotherapists. On average, effective interventions had a more diverse team of healthcare professionals than non-effective interventions. In addition, occupational therapists and physiotherapists were a standard part in most of the effective interventions (Buma et al, 2022). An explanation for this might be that in a diverse team there is a broader base of knowledge, skills and resources available, allowing various viewpoints to be applied on a problem.

Using the multiple components of reablement – among them, participation in daily activities and physical exercises – requires professional competence in facilitating, adjusting, and grading these components related to the health condition and progress of that person. It also requires the right attitude of 'doing with' instead of 'doing to', and although this may seem straightforward, it can conflict with the basic learning from the training that the professionals have received, that is, always to help and assist. Applying the right professional competencies and cultural mindset is particularly important for individuals with complex needs (Eliassen et al, 2018). Occupational therapists and physiotherapists are therapy personnel well equipped for facilitating the application of reablement training elements. However, other health and social-care workers may also assist after instruction and may even take the leading role on a daily basis (see, for instance, Rostgaard and Graff, 2016). In addition, other health- and social care personnel may provide a social dimension to the reablement intervention; for instance, in understanding how support from family members and third sector may be important. However, with increasing team size, the complexity of interdisciplinary collaboration also increases, emphasising the importance of having a team coordinator (Buma et al, 2020).

Regular assessments

In order to follow the progress and continuously adapt the intervention to the older individual's present status and to perhaps modify goals, as is often the case in rehabilitation, there must be regular assessments of the individual's functional capacities. Assessment can be formally carried out by a need assessor or a therapist, or it can be a more informal consideration incorporated into the daily practice of the reablement care worker.

Staff training

Success in reablement is dependent on staff training. A scoping review on reablement models of staff training found that reablement programmes are not yet embedded as a framework for standard practice by service providers in primary care settings (Bramble et al, 2022). Different programmes of training have been designed based on single disciplinary approaches and the context in which they are offered. Four reablement training programmes in the review contained an educational, theoretical component in combination with a more hands-on component, while four other studies comprised an educational component with a role-play or simulation element attached. Each training programme was initiated by one allied health professional or a nurse and tailored to reablement care/support worker with the aim for them to better understand and apply the principles of reablement, support clients in behaviour change, build better relationships with clients and increase knowledge and skills in reablement practices (Bramble et al, 2022). Another review (Buma et al, 2022) found that staff training was related to care delivery (meaning use of goal-setting tools, assessment procedures and so on) in the form of lectures, seminars, courses, and education by members of the team.

The theoretical aspects of reablement

While it is important to understand how these model features in combination constitute *what is reablement*, there is an apparent lack of an underlying theory that allows us to consider, from a theoretical perspective, *how* and *why* it works (Whyte, 2014; Wade, 2015). In a systematic review of reablement studies, Legg et al (2016: 746) state that:

> There is no well-developed understanding of the problem that it is intended to address, and the intervention lacks any explicit conceptual or theoretical framework. There is no clearly defined theory of change or mechanisms by which a reablement intervention programme might achieve its intended outcomes.

In other words, the reablement approach has been criticised for lacking a clear understanding of what it was trying to solve and what was the key to success. Thuesen et al (2021) attempt to counter this argument by considering the key principles, components and outcomes in reablement within a sociocultural theoretical approach to successful ageing that considers medical, epidemiological, and psychological aspects. However, it is also important to consider a wider perspective of the fundamental theoretical foundations of reablement. An important consideration is the considerable work published over the past 10–15 years around the need to ground the practice of rehabilitation within solid theoretical models (McPherson et al, 2015; Wade, 2015; Wade, 2016).

As the chapters in this book give evidence to, one fact that complicates any discussion of theories of reablement is that, similar to rehabilitation, reablement is a hybrid discipline in many respects. The theoretical roots of reablement lie partly in the various parent disciplines of which it is comprised, such as medicine, social work and social policy, gerontology, nursing, occupational therapy, and physiotherapy. Moreover, each of these parent disciplines draws upon other disciplines for its own theoretical foundations.

This requires a close exploration of the theories underpinning reablement at a grand, meta-range, mid-range and micro-range level (see Figure 2.1). At the *grand theory level*, it is important to consider both the system and the community perspective on the dominant paradigm that drives health and social care. Grand theory considers major paradigms, conceptual models and frameworks and covers fundamental world views and assumptions. This level includes *positivism* (knowledge and truth are considered as objective notions verified by the empirical sciences) and *post-positivism* (questions basic assumptions in positivism, for instance proposing that knowledge is not based on unchallengeable, rock-solid foundations, but rather human conjectures) and *interpretivism* (truth and knowledge are subjective and culturally and historically situated).

In addition, at the grand theory level there are concepts such as *liberalism* (that takes protecting and enhancing individual freedom to be the central issue in society) through to *institutionalism* (that emphasise the role of institutions in shaping and driving behaviour in society). Consideration of these concepts allows for critical reflection on the emphasis placed on different aspects of reablement models (such as a focus on independence, the importance of person–centred goal setting, and the need to manage costs and minimise health and social care expenditure).

When considering reablement within a country or more local context, it is important to be aware of the impact of the relevant dominance of grand theories on the planning, delivery, and evaluation of the service. The success factors and the philosophy underlying the reablement model may be significantly influenced by these fundamental concepts. An example is that

Figure 2.1: Overview of the theories underpinning reablement at a grand, meta-range, mid-range, and micro-range level

Grand level	Meta-range level	Mid-range level	Micro-range level
Both the system and the community perspective on the *dominant paradigm* that trives health and social care	Models and theories relating to ageing, which can help us identify the *understanding of the problem*	Identify *what drives and motivates clients* for developing functional capacity	Explore *change mechanisms* as to how and why interventions have an impact on the individual client
Positivism	Active ageing	Governmentality	Treatment theory
Postpositivism	Successful ageing	Empowerment	Enablement theory
Interpretivism			
Liberalism			
Institutionalism			

the understanding of what is proper evidence for the success of reablement may rely on the assumption that only RCT-based investigations are valid. Or that reablement may challenge a liberal notion that the individual knows best.

At the *meta-range level of theory*, it is important to consider theories relating to ageing, which can help us identify the *understanding of the problem*, as expressed for instance, in politics and policy. Reablement sits well within the dominant paradigm of *active ageing* (Thuesen et al, 2021) as it offers a platform with new individual and institutional means of action to displace the former 'decline and loss paradigm' (Holstein and Minkler, 2007: 787). The active ageing theory supports the continuation of regular activities, roles, and social relations, also in old age, from the hypothesis that activity and engagement contribute to a higher quality of life, as well as longer lives (Havighurst, 1961). A similar approach is found in the theory of *successful ageing* as formulated by Rowe and Kahn (1997), which outlined active engagement as one of the three pillars for achieving successful ageing in combination with a low degree of disability and illness and a high physical and cognitive functional capacity (see also Thuesen et al, 2021, and Chapter 1 by Rostgaard et al).

Addressing theories at the *mid-range level* can help us identify *what drives and motivates clients* for developing functional capacity. Depending on the theoretical starting point, such theories may vary. A *governmentality* perspective would, for instance, point to the processes of neoliberal responsibilisation and individualisation which implicitly force the individual to become responsible for help-to-self-help (Bødker et al, 2019; Clotworthy, 2020). From the perspective of behavioural theories, in particular *empowerment*, Empowerment Theory would point at the importance of engagement (Zimmerman and Warschausky, 1998), motivation (Siegert and Taylor, 2004), and behaviour change (Ajzen, 1991).

At the *micro-range level*, relevant theories for reablement may explore *change mechanisms* as to how and why interventions have an impact on the individual client. In the field of rehabilitation, micro-level theories may include *Treatment Theory* (Keith and Fuhrer, 1997), which specifies the more exact and active ingredients (practice and modification of a task, goal-setting, or environmental adaptation), and how they produce a change in the patient/client outcome. For example, as presented earlier, goal-setting has been shown to affect various aspects of human performance across many settings, including reablement, and may enhance the impact of treatments that aim to change complex human behaviours. Likewise, *Enablement Theory* (Whyte et al, 2014) may look beyond the bodily impairment and also address what other areas were affected as a result of reablement intervention and whether the treatment has the broader functional and participation effects the individual was hoping to achieve.

It is important to clearly acknowledge how theories from different disciplines and at different levels are applied and utilised within reablement research and practice as a universal reference point; doing so will assist with the interpretation and analysis of the effect and impact of reablement services. Acknowledging how the theories may have influenced the conceptualisation, design, delivery, and analysis of a reablement service is important. Equally important is the effect of the different levels of theory on the end-user of the research, whether these are practitioners, policy makers, clients, or others. This is shown clearly in a number of the chapters in this book in which the outcomes used to define success for a reablement intervention varies considerably. Attempts to unpack what may or may not be successful components of reablement are in their infancy, but the content of this book clearly illustrates where some of this work could be focused.

Conclusion

This chapter has presented a comparative perspective on main regional characteristics of the four different regions covered in the book: Australasia (Australia and New Zealand), Scandinavia (Denmark, Norway, and Sweden), and western (England) and central Europe (the Netherlands). These are all ageing societies with more than 15 per cent of the populations aged 65+ and average life expectancies well over 80 years. Despite their placement in different welfare regimes, they have all introduced reablement, and as shown in the presentation of the institutional characteristics, there is some similarity across the seven countries in the approach to reablement. Also, they generally apply what can be considered the main model features, which are unique to the reablement approach. As presented in the chapter these reablement model features are the following: Reablement is often targeted a home-dwelling older adults. It is a holistic intervention with several components. In fact, effective reablement interventions include multiple components. The interdisciplinary teams often consist of reablement care/support workers, registered nurses, occupational therapists, and physiotherapists, and effective interventions have a diverse team of healthcare professionals. The intervention should be relation-based, intensive and of short duration, as shorter durations are more effective. Focus on person-centredness and goal-setting are essential features of the intervention. It is vital that reablement takes place in a familiar context where the client lives. It is also important that regular assessments are applied and that staff involved are being offered training.

While the application of these model features can explain why the reablement intervention may be successful, as argued in the chapter, it is also essential to understand the theoretical framework behind reablement and how this on various levels may support the application of reablement. The theoretical roots of reablement lie partly in the various parent disciplines of which it is comprised. Grand theory considers major paradigms, conceptual models, and frameworks, and covers fundamental world views and assumptions. At the meta-range level of theory, reablement sits well within the dominant paradigm of active ageing as it offers a platform with new individual and institutional means of action to displace the former 'decline and loss' paradigm. Finally, at the micro-range level, relevant theories for reablement may explore *change mechanisms* as to how and why interventions have an impact on the individual client.

Acknowledgements

We would like to thank the members of the ReAble Network for input regarding the cross-country analysis of the seven countries.

Note

[1]   England is used to exemplify the United Kingdom, as there is most information from this country.

References

Ajzen, I. (1991) 'The theory of planned behavior', *Organizational Behavior and Human Decision Processes*, 50(2): 179–211.

Aspinal, F., Glasby, J., Rostgaard, T., Tuntland, H., and Westendorp, R. (2016) 'New horizons: reablement – supporting older people towards independence', *Age and Ageing*, 45(5): 574–8.

Azim, F.T., Burton, E., Ariza-Vega, P., Asadian, M., Bellwood, P., Burns J., et al (2022) 'Exploring behavior change techniques for reablement: a scoping review', *Brazilian Journal of Physical Therapy*, 26(2): 100–401.

Bergström, A., Vik, K., Haak, M., Metzelthin, S., Graff, L., and Hjelle, K.M. (2022) 'The jigsaw puzzle of activities for mastering daily life: service recipients and professionals' perceptions of gains and changes attributed to reablement – A qualitative meta-synthesis', *Scandinavian Journal of Occupational Therapy*, 1–12.

Birkeland, A., Tuntland, H., Førland, O., Jacobsen, F., and Langeland, E. (2017) 'Interdisciplinary collaboration in reablement – a qualitative study', *Journal of Multidisciplinary Healthcare*, 10: 195–203.

Bødker, M., Christensen, U., and Langstrup, H. (2019) 'Home care as reablement or enabling arrangements? An exploration of the precarious dependencies in living with functional decline', *Sociology of Health & Illness*, 41(5): 1358–72.

Bramble, M., Young, S., Prior, S., Maxwell, H., Campbell, S., Marlow A., et al (2022) 'A scoping review exploring reablement models of training and client assessment for older people in primary health care', *Primary Health Care Research & Development*, 23: e11.

Buma, L., Vluggen, S., Zwakhalen, S., Kempen, I.J.M, and Methzelthin, S.F. (2022) 'Effects on clients' daily functioning and common features of reablement interventions: a systematic literature review', *European Journal of Ageing*. DOI: 10.1007/s10433-022-000693-3

Chiu, E.-C., Chi, F.-C., and Chen, P.-T. (2021) 'Investigation of the home-reablement program on rehabilitation outcomes for people with stroke: a pilot study', *Medicine*, 100(26): e26515.

Clotworthy, A. (2020) *Empowering the Elderly? How 'Help to Self-help' Interventions Shape Ageing and Eldercare in Denmark*, Bielefeld, Germany: Transcript Verlag (Aging Studies series XX).

Clotworthy, A., Kusumastuti, S., and Westendorp, R. (2021) 'Reablement through time and space: a scoping review of how the concept of "reablement"' for older people has been defined and operationalised', *BMC Geriatrics*, 21(1): 1–16.

Eliassen, M., Henriksen, N., and Moe, S. (2018) 'The practice of support personnel, supervised by physiotherapists, in Norwegian reablement services', *Physiotherapy Research International*, e1754.

Elissen, A.M.J., Verhoeven, G.S., de Korte, M.H., van den Bulck, A.O.E., Metzelthin, S., van der Weij, L., Stam, J., Ruwaard, D., and Mikkers, M.C. (2020) 'Development of a casemix classification to predict costs of home care in the Netherlands: a study protocol', *BMJ Open*, 10(2): e035683.

Fisher, A.G. and Marterella, A. (2019) *Powerful Practice: A Model for Authentic Occupational Therapy*, Fort Collins, Colorado: Ciots.

Havighurst, R.J. (1961) 'Successful aging', *The Gerontologist*, 1: 8–13.

Hjelle, K., Tuntland, H., Førland, O., and Alvsvåg, H. (2016) 'Driving-forces for home-based reablement: a qualitative study of older adults' experiences', *Health & Social Care in the Community*, 1–9.

Holstein, M.B. and Minkler, M. (2007) 'Critical gerontology: reflections for the 21st century', *Critical Perspectives on Ageing Societies*, 13–26.

Keith, R. and Fuhrer, M. (1997) *The Role of Treatment Theory. Assessing Medical Rehabilitation Practices: The Promise of Outcomes Research*, Baltimore, MD: Paul H. Brookes Publishing Co.

Langeland, E., Tuntland, H., Folkestad, B., Førland, O., Jacobsen, F., and Kjeken, I. (2019) 'A multicenter investigation of reablement in Norway: a clinical controlled trial', *BMC Geriatrics*, 19(29). DOI: 10.1186/s12877-019-1038-x

Law, M., Baptiste, S., Carswell, A., McColl, M., Polatajko, H., and Pollock, N. (2015) *COPM Canadian Occupational Performance Measure (Norwegian Version)*, Oslo: NKRR National Advisory Unit on Rehabilitation in Rheumatology.

Legg, L., Gladman, J., Drummond, A., and Davidson, A. (2016) 'A systematic review of the evidence on home care reablement services', *Clinical Rehabilitation,* 30(8): 741–9.

McGormack, B., McCance, T., and Klopper, H. (2017) '*Person-Centred Practice in Nursing and Health Care: Theory and Practice*', West Sussex: Wiley Blackwell.

McPherson, K.M., Kayes, N.M. and Kersten, P. (2015) 'Meaning as a smarter approach to goals in rehabilitation', in R.J. Siegert and W. Levack (ed) *Handbook of Rehabilitation Goal Setting*, San Francisco: CRC Press/Taylor & Francis, pp 105–19.

Metzelthin, S., Rostgaard, T., Parsons, M., and Burton, E. (2020) 'Development of an internationally accepted definition of reablement: a Delphi study', *Ageing and Society*, 42(3): 703–18.

Mulquiny, L. and Oakman, J. (2022) 'Exploring the experience of reablement: a systematic review and qualitative evidence synthesis of older people's and carers' views', *Health & Social Care in the Community*, 1–13.

Newton, C. (2012) 'Personalising reablement: inserting missing link', *Working with Older People*, 16(3): 117–21.

OECD (2019) *Health at a Glance 2017: OECD Indicators*, OECD Publishing.

OECD (nda) *Health At a Glance 2021*. OECD Stat [online], Available from: https://www.oecd.org/health/health-at-a-glance/

OECD (ndb) *Health Status*. OECD Stat [online], Available from: https://stats.oecd.org/index.aspx?DataSetCode=HEALTH_STAT

OECD (ndc) *Long-Term Care Resources and Utilisation*. OECD Stat [online], Available from: https://stats.oecd.org/Index.aspx?DataSetCode=HEALTH_LTCR

ONS (nd) 'Changes in the older resident care home population between 2001 and 2011', Office for National Statistics [online], Available from: https://www.ons.gov.uk/peoplepopulationandcommunity/birthsdeathsandmarriages/ageing/articles/changesintheolderresidentcarehomepopulationbetween2001and2011/2014-08-01#:~:text=At%20age%2065%20and%20over,resident%20population%3B%20see%20table%201

Parsons, J.G.M. and Parsons, M.J.G. (2012) 'The effect of a designated tool on person-centred goal identification and service planning among older people receiving homecare in New Zealand', *Health & Social Care in the Community*, 20(6): 653–62.

Parsons, M., Rouse, P., Sajtos, L., Harrison, J., Parsons, J., and Gestro, L. (2018) 'Developing and utilising a new funding model for homecare services in New Zealand', *Health & Social Care in the Community*, 26(3): 345–55.

Ranci, C. and Rostgaard, T. (eds) (forthcoming) *Research Handbook of Social Care Policy*, Cheltenham: Edward Elgar Publishing.

Rostgaard, T. and Graff, L. (2016) *Med hænderne i lommen – Borger og medarbejders samspil og samarbejde i rehabilitering*, VIVE report. Copenhagen: VIVE [online], Available from: https://www.vive.dk/da/udgivelser/med-haenderne-i-lommen-8841/

Rowe, J.W. and Kahn, R.L. (1997) 'Successful aging', *The Gerontologist*, 37(4): 433–40.

Siegert, R.J. and Taylor, W.J. (2004) 'Theoretical aspects of goal-setting and motivation in rehabilitation', *Disability and Rehabilitation*, 26(1): 1–8.

Thuesen, J., Feiring, M., Doh, D., and Westendorp, R. (2021) 'Reablement in need of theories of ageing: would theories of successful ageing do?', *Ageing & Society*, 1–13. DOI: 10.1017/S0144686X21001203

Tuntland, H., Kjeken, I., Langeland, E., Folkestad, B., Espehaug, B., Førland, O., and Aaslund, M. (2017) 'Predictors of outcomes following reablement in community-dwelling older adults', *Clinical Intervention in Aging*, 2017(12): 55–63.

Tuntland, H., Kjeken, I., Folkestad, B., Førland, O., and Langeland, E. (2019) 'Everyday occupations that older adults participating in reablement prioritise: a cross-sectional study', *Scandinavian Journal of Occupational Therapy*. DOI: 10.1080/11038128.2019.1604800

UN (2019) *World Population Ageing. Highlights*, NY: United Nations.

Wade, D. (2015) 'Rehabilitation – a new approach. Part two: the underlying theories', *Clinical Rehabilitation*, 29(12): 1145–54.

Wade, D. (2016) 'Rehabilitation – a new approach. Part three: the implications of the theories', *Clinical Rehabilitation*, 30(1): 3–10.

Wade, D., Smeets, R.J., and Verbunt, J.A. (2010) 'Research in rehabilitation medicine: methodological challenges', *Journal of Clinical Epidemiology*, 63(7): 699–704.

Whyte, J. (2014) 'Contributions of treatment theory and enablement theory to rehabilitation research and practice', *Archives of Physical Medicine and Rehabilitation*, 95(1): S17–S23.e2.

Whyte, J., Dijkers, M.P., Hart, T., Zanca, J.M., Packel, A., Ferraro, M., and Tsaousides, T. (2014) 'Development of a theory-driven rehabilitation treatment taxonomy: conceptual issues', *Archives of Physical Medicine and Rehabilitation*, 95(1): S24–S32.e2.

World Health Organization (2015) 'WHO global strategy on people-centred and integrated health services: interim report', World Health Organization [online], Available from: https://apps.who.int/iris/handle/10665/155002

World Health Organization (nd) 'The Global Health Observatory', [online], Available from: www.who.int

Zimmerman, M.A. and Warschausky, S. (1998) 'Empowerment theory for rehabilitation research: Conceptual and methodological issues', *Rehabilitation Psychology*, 43(1): 3.

3

The ideas of reablement and their travel across time and space

Marte Feiring, Oddvar Førland, Fiona Aspinal, and Tine Rostgaard

Introduction

Across a number of regions, the overall approach and design of reablement services were originally objectified under different names when they were enacted, and sometimes, institutionalised, in different geographical contexts. Nevertheless, there is a striking resemblance in the ideas of reablement and how they have materialised into reablement policies and practices, with common elements across regional locations and in specific countries (Metzelthin et al, 2020).

This chapter investigates the travelling of these ideas and their materialisation into reablement policies and practices, internationally as well as nationally. The main analysis explores whether and how the ideas behind reablement have travelled within and across three regional empirical cases and materialised into national policies and local practices. The chapter also investigates how this development has been supported sequentially by the policy agendas of 'active and healthy ageing', which have been part of international policy rhetoric for years, by such organisations as the European Union (EU), Organisation of Economic Co-operation and Development (OECD), and World Health Organization (WHO).

Two theoretical frameworks are applied: the travel of ideas across localities (Czarniawska and Joerges, 1996), and rhetorical frames related to policy change (Béland, 2009). The chapter is organised in three sections: after the theoretical framework and research methods are presented, the development of the transnational ideas of active and healthy ageing is outlined, and how these ideas may have materialised into objects and contributed to local actions and national institutions in three world regions are analysed; the chapter is rounded off with a discussion and a conclusion.

This study illustrates how ideas and local processes behind enabling and active approaches to ageing have not been unidirectional but rather a set of complex and composite processes. In many countries, there have been significant bottom-up processes as practical responses to ageing populations and financial pressures on public services; as we see it, however, influenced by the transnational ideas of active and healthy ageing.

Theoretical perspectives

To analyse these processes of travelling ideas, the chapter mainly draws on Barbara Czarniawska and her co-writers' study of organisational changes across localities (Czarniawska and Joerges, 1996). The travelling ideas concept is understood as referring to 'processes of translation' or the sense that 'to set something in a new place is to construct it anew' (Latour, 1987, as cited in Czarniawska and Sevón, 2005: 8). They claim that similar policy and practice changes are often introduced at about the same time in different localities, and 'that all ideas circulate most of the time, at least in some places' (Czarniawska and Joerges, 1996: 14). To identify these ideas in terms of images of communication, the authors recommend starting with narratives at a given moment and then tracing them through different localities and moments in global time and space. Following this method, the interest here is in how ideas are materialised, translated, and travel to new localities; for example, from local to national to international level – or the other way around. According to Czarniawska, to materialise an idea is to turn it into an 'object' (that is a text, picture, prototype) and onward into an 'action', repeated and stabilised, which is further embedded in an 'institution' (that is a routine, norm, or rule). This theoretical perspective enables the analysis of the translation of ideas of reablement into actual practices and how they have materialised in different geographical contexts (Czarniawska and Sevón, 2005).

We also utilise the work of Daniel Béland (2009) on political agenda-setting and his claim that ideas constitute a major component in the identification and construction of social problems that (do not) enter the policy agenda. Referring to Parsons (2002), Béland defines ideas as 'claims about descriptions of the world, causal relationships, or the normative legitimacy of certain actions' (Béland, 2009: 702). Following Béland, we apply the term 'rhetorical frames' to understand how discursive constructions of problems and their solutions often appeal to shared cultural understandings and serve as 'institutional blueprints' for problem identification and available solutions for national and local actors. The interest is particularly in how reablement replies to problem identifications, applying the rhetoric of active and healthy ageing at the local, national, and international levels, here drawing on how policy agendas of supranational organisations (that is OECD, WHO, EU) may have contributed to the materialisation of the ideas of reablement. The interest is not in how certain ideas came to dominate or which ideas were left behind; hence, we do not conduct a multi-stream analysis of the agenda-setting of ideas (Kingdon and Stano, 1984; as cited in Béland and

Howlett, 2016) but identify instead how the dominant and paradigmatic ideas constitute rhetorical frames for the travelling of reablement in local, regional, and international time and space. This travelling may have taken place in many ways and might involve travels within a country or between countries and regions over time.

Methods

We have selected three regional cases following a description and discussion of how different countries have approached reablement in the ReAble research network (ReAble Network – https://reable.auckland. ac.nz/). First, the United Kingdom (UK), which was most likely where the name 'reablement' was first used. Second, an Australasian case, where the ideas to establish restorative care may have come from supranational organisations and inspired Australia and New Zealand; and third, a Scandinavian case, where the reablement approach has travelled between the three Nordic countries, from Sweden to Denmark and Norway. The six countries share several characteristics; they are post-industrial, their policy environment has been strongly influenced by neo-liberal trends (most recently in the guise of new public governance), and their populations are growing rapidly (see also Chapter 2 by Tuntland et al). There are few prior comparisons about geographical trajectories of reablement, possibly because it is a relatively new approach to long-term care (LTC), the one exception is Lewin (2011).

Our empirical data comprise eight expert interviews and multiple national and international policy documents. Interviews were conducted in 2019, either face-to-face or via Skype, with key informants, all experts in the development of reablement within their region/country. The choice of informants was guided by consulting members of the ReAble research network. Interview guides were informed by the theoretical framework described previously. All the interviews were videotaped or recorded, transcribed, corrected, and analysed by the four researchers. These data were triangulated with websites, grey literature, and policy documents. All the data were examined following the Braun and Clarke (2020) thematic analysis method. The interviewees (named A–H) signed an informed consent agreement. One person from each region has read and agreed to the presentation of the cases.

The transnational travelling of ideas

From an international perspective, the ideas later materialising as reablement on regional and country levels have many forerunners. As a gerontological paradigm, reablement draws on the concept of successful ageing and the connection between activity and health (Thuesen et al, 2021). The ageing of populations in Western societies since the early 1990s sparked an interest in whether and how transformative changes in LTC policies could contribute to more preventive approaches that would keep costs down, and eventually improve quality of life. In the mid-1990s, for instance, the OECD identified ageing as a policy challenge and recommended active and productive ageing as a policy response for developed countries (OECD, 1994). Despite vagueness in the definition and conceptualisation of active ageing (Walker and Maltby, 2012), it has become a common policy discourse across pan-national governance agencies, including the WHO and EU (European Commission, 1999; WHO, 1999).

Despite the potential of this conceptualisation of active ageing, over time the EU policy focus on active ageing became primarily aligned with an economic/productivity concept centred on retaining an ageing workforce in employment (Walker and Maltby, 2012). In 2013, however, the European Commission also acknowledged the social and economic returns of considering an active approach to LTC in its social investment strategy (de la Porte and Natali, 2018). The Commission specifically singled out reablement and pointed to Danish reablement practices in the municipality of Fredericia, because they increased 'the possibility of raising the overall quality of protection against long-term care risks' (European Commission, 2013: 19). Thus, reablement is here perceived as a risk-minimisation policy strategy, protecting the individual against the risks and potential dependencies associated with ageing, as well as enabling welfare states to dynamically manage the societal risks associated with ageing populations.

Simultaneously, a discourse of healthy ageing with a particular focus on improving individual wellbeing became prominent. After a hiatus of this concept in WHO documents since 2002, the WHO returned to healthy ageing with its 2015 World Report on Ageing and Health, defining it as 'the process of developing and maintaining the functional ability that enables well-being in older age' (WHO, 2020: 1). According to the WHO framework, this functional ability is determined by the intrinsic capacity of the individual (the combination of the individual's physical and mental − including psychosocial − capacities), the environments they inhabit (understood in the broadest sense and including physical, social, and policy environments), and the interaction between them. As such, the approach creates a rhetorical framing of the need for an enabling policy framework focused on developing and maintaining the individual's capacity for daily functioning, which is therefore aligned with the reablement approach. The launch of the new WHO healthy ageing agenda took place at the International Federation of Ageing (IFA) Copenhagen Summit in 2015, which, for the first time, gathered international context experts and policymakers interested in the reablement approach as an innovative and new element in LTC. As stated in the concluding report, 'the reablement approach is part of a new narrative that challenges the negative discourse around ageing and age-related morbidities, offering instead a perspective that focuses on intrinsic capacity, functional ability and healthy ageing' (IFA Copenhagen and DaneAge, 2016: 31) and is thus closely aligned with WHO strategies.

In line with Béland's ideational framework of political agenda-setting and arguments for how ideas contribute to what is identified as a policy problem as well as their solution, supranational organisations are seen to have aligned themselves over time with and contributed to the discourse that LTC policy must support and enable the individual maintenance of functional ability (Bødker, 2018). This signifies a change in the understanding of the capacity of public policy to not only stall limitations in daily functioning, but also to help improve such functioning. In so doing, supranational organisations could contribute to the construction of a shared cultural understanding of what the problem is and how possible policy, practice, and individuals lead solutions to address functional decline. Viewed from the perspective of how ideas are translated across time and space, these supranational organisations may have contributed to the objectification of ideas underpinning reablement, such as active and healthy ageing, which can serve both as institutional blueprints for problem identification, and as the policy and practice solutions available to national and local actors. They may also have contributed to materialising these ideas into objects and actions by drawing on examples of existing national or local policies and reablement programmes, as witnessed with the EU Commission's case use of reablement in Fredericia, Denmark, to promulgate ideas underpinning reablement as well as the objects and actions associated with it.

Three regional cases

But is the international-to-national level problem identification really how reablement developed in our three case regions? And was reablement even a national initiative? This section outlines and compares whether and how ideas of active and healthy ageing travelled and were translated into concepts, activities/practices, and institutions of reablement across our case regions since the early 2000s. It also outlines whether developments drew on the international rhetorical frames of healthy and active ageing.

United Kingdom

Across all four UK nations (England, Northern Ireland, Scotland, and Wales), reablement developed in response to practical concerns about service demand and sustainability (acute health service demand, including hospital waiting times, 'bed blocking' and winter pressures, and increased demand for long-term social care) coupled with traction of the idea that short-term interventions could prevent or delay demand for LTC; and in so doing, optimise the cost-efficiency of the LTC system (Parker et al, 1999). Only more recently, the rhetorical reframing of the importance of short-term interventions for healthy and active ageing, and ageing-in-place has taken a central role in justifying continued reablement service expansion within and across the nations of the UK. Although the factors influencing service development were experienced across the UK, initiatives to counter these problems often arose in response to specific local organisational and demographic needs rather than via country – or indeed UK-wide – policy or practice responses. This resulted in variations in reablement practices and models within and across UK countries.

England was the first country in the UK to develop reablement services (Cowpe, 2005; Clotworthy et al, 2020) with the earliest LTC reablement service being a pilot service in Leicestershire that began in 2000 (Interview A). Around the same time, other services with a similar remit – 'intermediate care' and reablement – were already in place or developing in other parts of England. Contemporaneously, nation-level health and social care policy discourses began emphasising the importance of services supporting people to maximise their potential (Department of Health, 1998) and identified the new service delivery approaches, such as more health-related intermediate care, which was primarily aimed at reducing the demand for acute care provision (Secretary of State for Health, 2000) (Interviews B and C). Rapid growth in intermediate care services, which were predominantly led by health organisations, was seen following substantial financial support being made available. At the same time, local authority social services departments were developing reablement services to address similar concerns with reducing demand for LTC. A survey of local councils across England conducted by the Department of Health Care Services Efficiency Delivery Programme in 2004, helped to identify a new approach – reablement – for providing home care in a handful of local councils. These services seem to have developed independently of each other, were geographically distanced, and were in demographically different areas. According to the interviewee, local managers agreed that their services developed in response to local demographic changes and service demand, rather than ideological paradigms or policy initiatives (Interview A). Since 2004, there has been a huge expansion of reablement service provision across England but with little evidence about best practice to inform service development, there was, and remains, wide variation in service delivery models (Beresford et al, 2019). Increasingly blurred lines between health-led intermediate care and social care-led reablement, as services respond to the policy demand for more integrated provision, has only exacerbated this variation. Explaining with certainty why individual reablement services developed in a particular way since 2004 is difficult, but our empirical data suggests that similar to the earlier examples, they did so in response to local needs and structures, with wider policy initiatives and discourses only having an influence more latterly.

Reablement services developed in *Wales* in the early 2000s, and similar to other UK nations, these initiatives were often locally driven, resulting in a complex mix of delivery mechanisms, ranging from dedicated reablement teams to being one element of integrated community provision, something that can, in part, be explained by the Government making money available to enhance intermediate care services (SSIA, 2016). Nevertheless, the distinction between intermediate care and reablement, which has now become blurred across other UK nations, remains intact in Welsh documents where reablement continues to be presented as a social care, rather than an integrated or health model (Age Cymru, 2019). While legislation in Wales has led to conformity in, for example, the approach to eligibility, variation in service composition, level of integration, and aims of services, continues.

The first reablement service in *Scotland* was established in Edinburgh in 2008 as a mechanism for reducing the need for LTC. This was quickly followed by other locally led initiatives, including in Glasgow and North Lanarkshire. Based on a government-commissioned evaluation that documented significant increases in efficiency (41 per cent reduction in home care hours required post reablement), reablement was endorsed as a short-term care model to help reduce the demand for LTC (McLeod and Mair, 2011). As in England, the dominant ideas driving reablement expansions across Scotland remain focused on cost-efficiency (COSLA et al, 2011). While later texts also emphasise the importance of self-determination and optimising independence in line with healthy ageing concepts, evaluations continue to report results related to service use prevention rather than measures of independence. Like the English experience, boundaries between intermediate care and reablement have blurred, with intermediate care being increasingly viewed as an umbrella term for short-term prevention interventions for people in their homes including reablement (NICE, 2018).

In *Northern Ireland*, reablement was first proposed following a review of care (Northern Ireland Assembly, 2011), and the five Health and Social Care Trusts (HSCT) across Northern Ireland started developing and expanding reablement services in 2012, using a planned approach for delivery. Northern Ireland, with this nationally led approach and national guidelines to inform reablement delivery, is therefore distinct from the rest of the UK, where reablement originated in small pockets, led by key champions in response to local challenges and without nationally agreed definitions or guidance on delivery approaches. Nevertheless, despite guidance about eligibility, service delivery, and evaluation, a service audit in 2014 indicated diversity in how the reablement guidance had been interpreted locally and how services were delivered across Northern Ireland (Health & Social Care Board, 2015). To maximise consistency across HSCTs, new guidance documents endorsed an expanded scope of reablement services, clarified reablement service leadership, and outlined how services should be accessed and delivered (Health & Social Care Board, 2015); nevertheless, it remains unclear whether this has reduced variation across the reablement environment in Northern Ireland. The national interest in reablement illustrated in these national documents and each HSCT's apparent commitment to reablement provision indicate that reablement has become a normalised component of HSCT provision for older adults.

Looking across the four UK nations, except for Northern Ireland, the reablement services in LTC were primarily initiated by key professionals viewing existing care arrangements as unsustainable in the light of changing local demographics and associated demand (Interview A). In short, these were bottom-up initiatives driven by local champions. Policy lagged behind the practice and, although reablement is now a recognised approach through which local councils can reduce dependency and prevent deterioration (Care Act, 2014: c. 23), variations remain in what is provided, its purpose, how it is provided, and who can access it. The primacy of efficiency and sustainability in driving reablement development is clear, but professionals were also enticed by the idea that these changes would also promote independence. These variations in models continue, and without evidence about the relative efficacy of different models for diverse client groups being established, they are likely to persist. Only latterly in reablement travels within and across the UK nations were conceptual discourses (for example active ageing) used as a justification or driver for change.

Australasia

As is generally the case in the UK, reablement was a response to the increasing need for long-term care in Australasia (Australia and New Zealand), but countries in this region seem to have drawn on the rhetorical frames of active and healthy ageing at an earlier stage in their development trajectory. In both countries, the introduction of the reablement approach also went hand in hand with the general development of ageing-in-place home care services as an alternative to more costly institutional care. Some differences were also evident, as Australia took a bottom-up approach, while national policies paved way for reablement in New Zealand.

In *Australia*, restorative home care, as reablement was first called there, was introduced by a 'professional entrepreneur' as a service activity in Perth in 1999 by Silver Chain, a large non-profit home care agency in Western Australia. The first restorative care practice, the Home Independence Program was, according to initiator Gill Lewin, a direct response to an increasing need for home care services (Lewin et al, 2006; Lewin, 2011). The new service was designed to help older citizens optimise their functioning and improve health conditions, thereby reducing the demand for residential care. The restorative care programme was time-limited, goal-directed, and delivered by a multidisciplinary health team of occupational therapists, physiotherapists, and nurses, in addition to trained reablement care workers (Lewin and Vandermeulen, 2008) (Interview D).

The new approach to ageing was soon manifested in national policy documents: 'The National Strategy for Ageing Australia' (2001) and later the 'New Strategy for Community Care – The Way Forward' (2004), all of which occurred several years before the first research in 2006 could establish that the approach was successful (Lewin et al, 2006; Lewin and Vandermeulen, 2010). After evidence of the effectiveness was established, the restorative home care services gradually travelled to other Australian states, and similar approaches were established in Victoria and New South Wales (Lewin, 2011). The new practices were all framed in the rhetoric of active ageing and wellness: including the active service model (Victoria), active consumer participation, and the Northern Sidney Wellness and Restorative project (New South Wales) (Cartwright, 2009). According to Lewin et al (2016) many home care agencies did not adopt the new model. Despite this lack of general adoption, there was increasing policy backing at the national level (Interview D). This included the national forum for home and community services in Melbourne (2008) with more than 400 participants. Five years later, a *National Primary Health Care Strategy* was launched, followed by a Short-Term Restorative Care Programme – an expansion of the Transition Care Programme for hospital discharge and the Commonwealth Home Support Programme (CHSP) – a comprehensive home support programme for older people aimed at training them to be able to remain in their home and community longer (Department of Health, 2013, 2015a, 2015b; Department of Social Services, 2015). The CHSP was funded by the federal, state, and territorial governments and the responsibility for all costs was transferred to the national level, and soon after the new Commonwealth Liberal-National Coalition Government proposed a revised model for reablement services (Interview D).

At about the same time as Western Australia, reablement was on the agenda in *New Zealand* but under the name 'restorative home support'. Initially, it was mainly intended to develop ageing-in-place services. In New Zealand, home support services were primarily delivered by non-government organisations, while the national government funded the needs assessments and service coordination via the District Health Boards (DHBs) (Weir, 2018). In contrast to the UK and Australia, the active ageing approach was first undertaken in New Zealand at the national, political level. The introduction of restorative home support was preceded by three new national policy programmes that were to frame the national policies on aged and disability care. Here, the vision was to develop new services that would strengthen the ability of the elderly to continue living in their own homes (Ministry of Social Development Office for Senior Citizens, 2001; Ministry of Health, 2002). This followed the 'ageing-in-place' slogan and included several projects funded through local and central authorities.

While national policies paved the way for the introduction of restorative care/reablement, entrepreneurs argue that the approach adopted in New Zealand also drew inspiration and evidence from the US and the UK (Interview E). The first restorative home care practice in New Zealand was named Community FIRST and implemented in 2002 in Auckland. It was one of three so-called ageing-in-place pilot initiatives from the Ministry of Health and DHBs, in collaboration with Auckland University and the Presbyterian Church. The aim was to promote independence and recovery among older citizens by applying a holistic, flexible, and inclusive approach. The services were delivered in senior citizens' homes via a flexible restorative support team of registered nurses, physiotherapists, and occupational therapists, in addition to supporting workers or therapy aids. In contrast to the reablement services in the UK and Australia, restorative home support in New Zealand has no time limits. The ideological framing of the approach drew on the active ageing rhetoric in aiming to improve the ability of older people (Ministry of Social Development Office for Senior Citizens, 2001). The ageing-in-place initiatives were all positively evaluated (Parsons et al, 2006) and restorative home support services travelled to other districts and regions in New Zealand from about 2004 (Interview E).

Later, the New Zealand Health Strategy and the Healthy Ageing Strategy replaced earlier policies (Ministry of Health, 2016a). The new vision was: 'All New Zealanders live well, stay well, get well, in a system that is people-powered, provides services closer to home, is designed for value and high performance, and works as one team in a smart system' (Ministry of Health, 2016b: 1). Drawing on rhetorics of enablement and participation, the new restorative care/reablement services also led to an associated shift in the funding structure and were generally seen as an effective response to major issues in the national home support sector, including high staff turnover and inefficient funding models (Interview E).

Scandinavia

The Scandinavian countries, Sweden, Denmark, and Norway are often seen as forerunners in the organisation of LTC services (Christensen and Wærness, 2018), with high levels of universal and affordable LTC compared to most other Western countries (see also Chapter 2 by Tuntland et al). For many years, and often as an inspiration from the international policy agenda, the rhetorical frames behind Scandinavian LTC policy have been an active ageing paradigm that rests on the idea that people should be able to perform daily activities and self-care as long as possible in their own homes and remain independent; so-called self-care (Interview H). In line with this, reablement has found a distinct area of impact in Scandinavia, even though there are differences across and within countries in how it is enacted and institutionalised. Especially Denmark and Norway have managed to roll out reablement on a larger or national level, and here with the particular potential for the sustainability of the LTC systems in mind.

In *Sweden*, like the rest of Scandinavia, the most common expression of this type of rehabilitation has been named 'everyday rehabilitation' (*vardagsrehabilitering*). The name originates from a home care project in the Swedish municipality of Östersund from around 1997. Here, physiotherapists and occupational therapists initiated close cooperation with the home care sector and district nurses, advising, supporting, and encouraging home-care client's training and efforts to improve their functioning in daily activities, rather than performing tasks for them. Östersund municipality experienced a positive response from the clients, staff, health managers, and politicians, and assessed lower costs for the home care services.

In the Scandinavian context, it is common to refer to this Swedish project as the first reablement service in the region. A vital entrepreneur in the early phase was Marita Månsson (Månsson, 2007), an occupational therapist, who later authored a book describing the concept. In this book, she also used the term 'home rehabilitation' (*vardagsrehabilitering*) for almost the same services. In Sweden, the term 'general rehabilitation' is also used to some extent. All these concepts are understood differently than specific and specialist rehabilitation – which demands more specific knowledge concerning human functions, diseases, injuries, treatment, and training carried out by healthcare professionals with specialist competence. Although Östersund was an early case, an extensive spread of reablement across Swedish municipalities did not occur – as it later did in Denmark and Norway (Interview F). However, the Swedish Association of Occupational Therapists coined this definition in 2014: 'Reablement is a rehabilitative approach, that encourages the elderly person to take action … to make use of the person's resources and opportunities to be active in everyday life' (Pettersson and Iwarsson, 2015: 7; authors' translation). In a Swedish government official report (2017), the term everyday rehabilitation is applied three times, claiming that it is becoming a matter of course in the care of older people (Swedish Government Official Report, 2017: 27, 35, 111). Unlike in Denmark and Norway, however, it has remained an ideal and has not resulted in organisational changes in how home care is provided and by which collaborating professions.

In *Denmark*, the establishment of reablement was first formally discussed around 2007, when a high-level meeting was arranged between the Danish

Union of Public Employees (FOA), the organisation for local government (KL), the DaneAge Association representing clients, and the Ministry of Health. The subject of the meeting was new approaches in LTC to pre-empt future challenges for the sustainability of the LTC system. With direct reference to the Östersund experiences, 'everyday rehabilitation' (*hverdagsrehabilitering*) was highlighted as a promising initiative. As such, this meeting can be viewed as pivotal for the start-up and early development of reablement for older people in Denmark.

Although this meeting can be considered a national initiative, reablement programmes were locally initiated, developed, and driven by singular municipalities (Interview G). The leading Danish municipality in the early phase was Fredericia. In 2006–2007, municipal representatives from Fredericia visited different municipalities in Norway and Sweden (including Östersund) to find inspiration for new and more active ways of providing home care. From this, they developed their reablement slogan: 'As Long as Possible in Your Own Life' (*Så længe som muligt i eget liv*) (Fredericia Kommune, nd). In 2008, Fredericia developed a trial of a short-term intensive physical training intervention called 'Everyday rehabilitation' as an alternative to traditional, compensatory home care. This emphasised skills mastery and support for self-care and independence. To emphasise the training element, the titles for the home care providers involved were changed to home-trainers and these work in close collaboration with occupational therapists and meet together regularly. A quantitative evaluation produced positive results, more satisfied employees, and the lower use of municipal care services, using a pre-post rather than an RCT design (Kjellberg and Ibsen, 2010; Kjellberg and Ibsen, 2011). Reablement was subsequently disseminated to other municipalities, which often developed variations of the Fredericia model, and often under a different name. Overall, the local programmes are promoted as active care, in this way drawing on the rhetorical activation framework. They are also often highlighted as ways of increasing the independence of the client and enhancing their quality of life. However, with the underlying goal to increase cost-effectiveness by containing the demand for home care (Rostgaard and Graff, 2016), the roll out has been accompanied by a stricter assessment for conventional and compensatory home care.

By 2013, 94 per cent of Danish municipalities had formalised reablement home programmes in place (Kjellberg et al, 2013). As one of our informants expressed: "It exploded within a few years, and it changed the long-term care services" (Interview G). This spread of reablement happened primarily from below, through local champions, without a distinct plan from either the national government or the organisation for local government, KL, but with general support across local politicians and trade unions representing social and healthcare workers and occupational and physiotherapists, while critical voices were raised by the nurses' trade union, the Danish Nurses

Organization, and the highly influential organisation that represented older people, the DaneAge Association. Since 2015 and by law, every municipality must offer a time-limited reablement intervention to home care applicants who have been assessed as having a so-called 'potential to improve their functional capacity' (Social Services Act, 2014, section 83a). Across the municipalities, the common term used today is rehabilitation.

While reablement comes under various local names in Denmark, in *Norway*, the most common term used has been and still is today 'Everyday rehabilitation'. Originally, the direct inspiration came from contact with Danish municipalities, especially the municipality of Fredericia, after 2010. The Norwegian Minister of Health and Care Services, alongside representatives from Norwegian municipalities, travelled to Denmark to learn from the experiences there. The Norwegian Association of Occupational Therapists played a key role during the first years after 2010, initiating and facilitating conferences and meetings with other Norwegian trade unions and associations, the Norwegian organisation for local and regional governments (KS), and other policymakers. The Ministry of Health and Care Services promised to support these initiatives financially if they included nurse and physiotherapist associations.

Norwegian municipalities started introducing reablement in 2011, first in small, then medium-sized, and finally in the larger municipalities. In 2019, three-quarters of all Norwegian municipalities had implemented some kind of reablement service (Rostad et al, 2020). There are several explanations for this rapid growth. Especially in the first years after 2010, entrepreneurs in the pioneer reablement municipalities expressed great fervour in conferences and through the rapidly growing reablement Facebook group established by Nils Erik Ness, the former president of the Association of Occupational Therapists (Interview H). Particular to the Norwegian approach has been the promotion of a slogan, 'What activities are important in your life now?', which was aimed at maintaining the focus on the individual client's goals and preferences.

In 2011, an official Norwegian Report, Innovation in the Care Services (NOU 2011 Committee, 2011: 11) was published and became a central policy document for Norwegian policymakers, together with Future Care, a government white paper (Ministry of Health and Care Services, 2012). These policy papers emphasised a restructuring of professional activities towards a sharper focus on prevention, early intervention, and the idea that rehabilitation must be a natural and central part of all care and nursing activity. In addition, both quantitative and qualitative research studies were initiated (Tuntland et al, 2015; Hjelle et al, 2016; Kjerstad and Tuntland, 2016) shortly after start-up, which soon indicated positive gains for both the clients and the municipal cost-savings potential. Although the results were few and ambiguous, this evidence played a role in the further implementation process. In the period 2013–2015, the Norwegian Directorate of Health gave grants to 43 municipalities to develop and implement reablement. This initiative was also evaluated (Langeland et al, 2016; Langeland et al, 2019) and legitimised further investment in reablement. Although the influence of cultural and structural factors seems to have had an impact, the growth, as in Denmark, primarily seems to represent a response to local challenges of cost-effectiveness and economic sustainability in the care services.

Case comparisons

We have thus far indicated how supranational organisations may have paved the way for ideas that later materialised into reablement and how the travels of reablement have taken place in localities situated within particular world regions.

Applying our theoretical concepts, Figure 3.1 illustrates how the ideas of active and healthy ageing may have travelled and circulated for decades in global, national and local spaces, contributing to problem and policy identification and implementation as well as in changes in professional practice. Like an idea whose time has come, the 'rhetorical frames' of active and healthy ageing seem to have inspired how reablement was translated into different 'objects' (for example policy texts, names of programs and schemes etc.), 'actions' (that is repeated services, ad hoc arrangements), and 'institutions' (that is routines, permanent services) (Czarniawska and Joerges, 1996; Béland, 2009). 'Objectified' into regional names such as 'intermediate care/reablement' (UK), 'restorative care/support' (Australasia), and 'home rehabilitation/everyday rehabilitation' (Scandinavia), the new approach was translated and enacted into local ad hoc services, mainly applying bottom-up strategies, initiated by professional entrepreneurs, and 'institutionalised' into entire care systems on a national level.

Despite common cultural influences and values across geographies, our country cases reveal only some consistency within a region and great variation across the regions. As for the travels within regions, various actions of reablement in health and social care services are identified across the four UK nations. Although as early as the mid-1990s, a new health service materialised as intermediate care was piloted, focusing on practical concerns such as bed-blocking, while the local governments responsible for social care services redesigned the home care reablement services, emphasising improving skills and capacities to assist independent living. In the UK case, intermediate care and reablement are practices that travelled from the local to the national level after a national initiative supporting local authorities to increase the efficiency of social care. The reablement approach travelled first to Wales (early 2000), a few years later to Scotland (2008), and finally to Northern Ireland (2011). Today, reablement is institutionalised as an

Figure 3.1: An illustration of how ideas of active and healthy ageing may have travelled

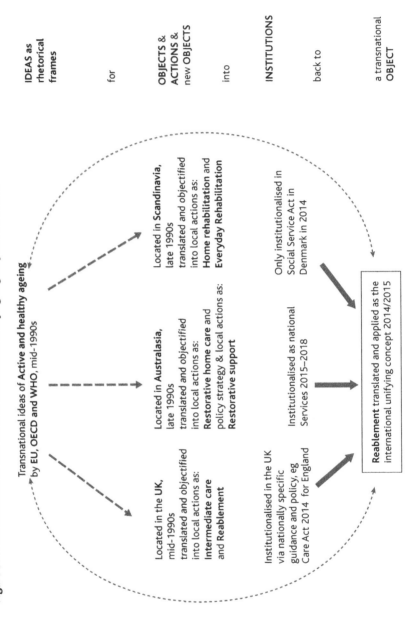

IDEAS as rhetorical frames

for

OBJECTS & ACTIONS & new OBJECTS

into

INSTITUTIONS

back to

a transnational OBJECT

Transnational ideas of **Active and healthy ageing** by **EU, OECD and WHO**, mid-1990s

Located in **Scandinavia**, late 1990s translated and objectified into local actions as: **Home rehabilitation** and **Everyday Rehabilitation**

Located in **Australasia**, late 1990s translated and objectified into local actions as: Restorative home care and policy strategy & local actions as: **Restorative support**

Located in the **UK**, mid-1990s translated and objectified into local actions as: **Intermediate care** and **Reablement**

Only institutionalised in Social Service Act in Denmark in 2014

Institutionalised as national Services 2015–2018

Institutionalised in the UK via nationally specific guidance and policy, eg Care Act 2014 for England

Reablement translated and applied as the international unifying concept 2014/2015

element of intermediate care in the NICE (2018) guidance in England and enshrined in national guidance and policy in each of the four nations and rhetorically framed as an active ageing service.

In Australia, the materialisation of a new active approach to ageing, termed restorative home care, was first introduced in Perth in Western Australia in 1999, initiated by a professional entrepreneur working in a large non-governmental organisation. The main aim was to reduce the demands for residential facilities for older citizens, and this new service activity was later translated into national policies (Lewin et al, 2006). New Zealand also located the first restorative home support in a populous city, Auckland, where several projects linked to the rhetorical ageing-in-place frame were initiated in 2002. A flexible and integrated restorative support team was addressed as the first ageing service to apply an active approach. Australia initiated the active service model referring to wellness as its foundation and applied a local-to-national strategy, while New Zealand developed an ageing-in-place policy slogan, piloting community participation first in national policy documents and from there to local pilot arrangements. Moreover, New Zealand was the only country in this study with an early reference to the rhetorical frameworks of the WHO and OECD and the ideas of active and healthy ageing (Parsons et al, 2017).

In Scandinavia, Sweden was the first country to initiate a reablement service in the late 1990s: an occupational therapist acted as an entrepreneur and expanded a rehabilitative approach to the older population in Östersund. This approach, first 'objectified' under the name 'home rehabilitation' and later 'everyday rehabilitation' did not develop throughout Sweden, travelling instead to the municipality of Fredericia in Denmark around 2007. From there, it was translated and enacted as a service throughout Denmark, where 'everyday rehabilitation' was 'institutionalised' and authorised by the Social Services Act in 2014. The rhetorical frame applied was to improve clients' independence and quality of life – but also achieve cost-efficiency. Norway looked both to Sweden and Denmark and initiated 'Everyday rehabilitation' services around 2011. As in Sweden, occupational therapists together with physiotherapists played the leading role, while the nurses were invited to join within a few years. The new approach was framed as person-centred and posed the question: 'What activities are important in your life now?' As in Denmark, the cost efficiency and future sustainability of long-term care was important rhetoric.

With one exception, New Zealand which was inspired by the US and UK, little travel of the idea of reablement is identified between the three regions. Instead, until the mid-2010s, our descriptions flesh out three rather separate regional processes of travelling that became enacted within the regions and are given an internationally unifying concept much later, not least by the development of the common Delphi-based definition of reablement as part of the ReAble Network activities (Metzelthin et al, 2020).

It is also evident that the initiatives were mainly local actions in an attempt to respond to ageing populations and financial pressure on public services, often without actual evidence of effectiveness and in several locations successfully promoted by individual entrepreneurs. The policy concerns generally seem to reflect the need for LTC sustainability and cost-efficiency. Regardless, the transnational ideas of active and healthy ageing have probably been part of common cultural values and are, therefore, indicated by the dotted line in Figure 3.1.

The three regional cases about the ideas of reablement and their travel indicate rather complex processes but with identifiable patterns. In our analysis, local practices mainly evolved as bottom-up processes objectified with different names and content. These local practices travelled in many directions and worked their way upwards into national politics and in some countries to whole-system care. This was the case in Australia, Denmark, England, Sweden, Scotland, and Wales. In contrast, the first service actions in New Zealand, Norway, and Northern Ireland were at the national level. Also in these countries, however, the main agenda seems to be the practical need to find more cost-effective policy solutions.

And common today for all regions and countries herein is that reablement practices are distinguishable actions that share common service elements such as goal-setting, regular assessments, and functional training by interdisciplinary teams in order 'to increase or maintain independence in a broad range of daily activities, including social, leisure or physical activities' (Metzelthin et al, 2020: 7).

Conclusion

In this study, we asked whether and how the ideas of active and healthy ageing have travelled, within regions and nations, inspired by individual or collective actors. Our analysis of regional cases indicates that reablement was mainly working its way from local initiatives and up before being objectified and materialised into ad hoc arrangements and later whole-system care. Only in three out of nine country cases was it from national to local level. The analysis supports the argument that the processes of travelling ideas and their materialisation are quite complex and composite and dependent on local and national factors.

We will sum up by indicating five processes: First, the ideational rhetoric of active and healthy ageing was not new in Western societies, but rather elements of common cultural values serving as 'frames' for identifying policy problems and their solutions. Second, what was new in the mid-1990s were the problems of a growing ageing population and the need for more sustainable and cost-efficient services. These practical concerns were identified early by supranational organisations and combined with dominant ageing paradigms of active and healthy ageing and constitute today's rhetorical frames for reablement at an international as well as national and local level. Third, in the late 1990s, these ideas were met with an often bottom-up initiated enabling approach to LTC, in many cases driven by individual entrepreneurs and champions or even particular trade unions, and resonating practical concerns related to sustainability and cost-efficiency of LTC in ageing societies. The ideas of active and healthy ageing later materialised into whole-system care and national regulations without being fully evidence-based but more reflecting that it was considered as a brilliant idea whose time had come. Fourth, the travels within and between regions illustrate that the notion of facilitating active and healthy ageing in reablement was originally 'objectified' and named differently across the three regions: intermediate care/reablement (UK), restorative care (Australasia), and home rehabilitation/everyday rehabilitation (Scandinavia) but share similar elements unique to the active reablement approach, including goal-setting, regular assessments, and functional training. Finally, these processes have culminated in the development of a generic definition of reablement for research purposes across the Western world and more importantly perhaps, the identification of the common model elements in the reablement approach, which have again triggered the interest of supranational organisations that now refer to reablement in their policy recommendations.

References

Age Cymru (2019) *Reablement, Intermediate Care and Preventative Services in Wales*, Cardiff: Age Cymru.

Béland, D. (2009) 'Ideas, institutions, and policy change', *Journal of European Public Policy*, 16(5): 701–18.

Béland, D. and Howlett, M. (2016) 'The role and impact of the multiple-streams approach in comparative policy analysis', *Journal of Comparative Policy Analysis: Research and Practice*, 18(3): 221–7.

Beresford, B., Mann, R., Parker, G., Kanaan, M., Faria, R., Rabiee, P., Weatherly, H., Clarke, S., Mayhew, E., Duarte, A., Laver-Fawcett, A., and Aspinal, F. (2019) 'Reablement services for people at risk of needing social care: the MoRe mixed-methods evaluation', *Health Services and Delivery Research*, 7(16).

Bødker, M.N. (2018) 'Potentiality made workable – exploring logics of care in reablement for older people', *Ageing & Society*, 39(9): 1–24.

Braun, V. and Clarke, V. (2020) 'One size fits all? What counts as quality practice in (reflexive) thematic analysis?', *Qualitative Research in Psychology*, 18(3): 328–52.

Care Act (2014) c. 23, London, UK Government, legislation.gov.uk.

Cartwright, C. (2009) *Re-ablement of Older People in North Coast, NSW, Australia*, New South Wales: South Cross University.

Christensen, K. and Wærness, K. (2018) 'Long-term care services in Norway: a historical sociological perspective', in K. Christensen and D. Pilling (eds), *The Routledge Handbook of Social Care Work Around the World*, Abingdon: Routledge, pp 15–28.

Clotworthy, A., Kusumastuti, S., and Westendorp, R. (2020) 'Reablement through time and space: a scoping review of how the concept of "reablement" for older people has been defined and operationalised', *BMC Geriatrics*, 21: 61.

COSLA, Scottish Government and NHS Scotland (2011) *Reshaping Care for Older People: A Programme for Change 2011–2021*, Edinburgh: The Scottish Government.

Cowpe, J. (2005) 'Intermediate care: policy and context', in B. Roe and R. Beech (eds), *Intermediate and Continuing Care: Policy and Practice*, New Jersey: Blackwell Publishing, pp 3–18.

Czarniawska, B. and Joerges, B. (1996) 'Travels of ideas', in B. Czarniawska-Joerges and G. Sevón (eds), *Translating Organizational Change*, Berlin: Walter de Gruyter, pp 13–48.

Czarniawska, B. and Sevón, G. (2005) *Global Ideas: How Ideas, Objects and Practices Travel in the Global Economy*, Stockholm: Liber & Copenhagen Business School Press.

de la Porte, C. and Natali, D. (2018) 'Agents of institutional change in EU policy: the social investment moment', *Journal of European Public Policy*, 25(6): 828–43.

Department of Health (1998) *Modernising Social Services (comnd 4169): Promoting Independence, Improving Protection, Raising Standards*, London: Stationery Office.

Department of Health (2013) *National Primary Health Care Strategic Framework*, Melbourne: Australian Government.

Department of Health (2015a) *Short-Term Restorative Care (STRC) Programme*, Canberra: Australian Government.

Department of Health (2015b) *Commonwealth Home Support Programme (CHSP) Guidelines Overview*, Canberra: Australian Government.

Department of Social Services (2015) *Living Well at Home – CHSP Good Practice Guide*, Canberra: Australian Government.

European Commission (1999) *New Paradigm in Ageing Policy*, Brussels: Employment and Social Affairs.

European Commission (2013) *Long Term Care in Ageing Societies – Challenges and Policy Options*, Brussels: Social Investment Package Commission.

Fredericia Kommune (nd) 'Længst Muligt i Eget Liv', Fredericia Kommune [online], Available from: https://www.fredericia.dk/borger/omsorg-sundhed/aeldreliv/laengst-muligt-i-eget-liv

Health & Social Care Board (2015) *Regional Reablement Model for Northern Ireland*, Belfast.

Hjelle, K.M., Tuntland, H., Førland, O., and Alvsvåg, H. (2016) 'Driving forces for home-based reablement: a qualitative study of older adults' experiences', *Health & Social Care in the Community*, 25(5): 1581-9.

IFA Copenhagen and DaneAge (2016) 'Final report: reablement and older people', [online], Available from: http://www.ifa-copenhagen-summit.com/wp-content/uploads/2016/04/Copenhagen-Summit-Final-Report.pdf

Kingdon, John W., and Eric Stano. 1984. Agendas, Alternatives, and Public Policies 45:165–69. London: Pearson Education.

Kjellberg, J. and Ibsen, R. (2010) *Økonomisk evaluering af Længst Muligt i Eget Liv i Fredericia Kommune*, Copenhagen: Dansk Sundhedsinstitut.

Kjellberg, J. and Ibsen, R. (2011) *Fra pleje og omsorg: viden og anbefalinger*, Copenhagen: Dansk Sundhedsinstitut.

Kjellberg, P.K., Hauge-Helgestad, A., Madsen, M.H., and Rasmussen, S.R. (2013) *Kortlægning af kommunernes erfaringer med rehabilitering på ældreområdet [Mapping of the Municipalities' Experiences with Reablement in the Eldercare Sector]*, Copenhagen: National Board of Social Services.

Kjerstad, E. and Tuntland, H.K. (2016) 'Reablement in community-dwelling older adults: a cost-effectiveness analysis alongside a randomized controlled trial', *Health Economics Review*, 6(1): 1–10.

Langeland, E., Førland, O., Aas, E., Birkeland, A., Folkestad, B., Kjeken, I., Jacobsen, F.F., and Tuntland, H. (2016) *Modeller for hverdagsrehabilitering – en følgeevaluering i norske kommuner*, Gjøvik: Senter for omsorgsforskning.

Langeland, E., Tuntland, H.K., Folkestad, B., Førland, O., Jacobsen, F.F., and Kjeken, I. (2019) 'A multicenter investigation of reablement in Norway: a clinical controlled trial', *BMC Geriatrics*, 19(29).

Latour, B. (1987) *Science in Action*, Cambridge, MA: Harvard University Press.

Lewin, G. (2011) 'Restorative home-care services', *Journal of Current Clinical Care*, 18(1): 91-9.

Lewin, G. and Vandermeulen, S. (2008) 'The Home Independence Project', *Geriaction*, 26(3): 13-20.

Lewin, G. and Vandermeulen, S. (2010) 'A non-randomised controlled trial of the Home Independence Program (HIP): an Australian restorative programme for older home-care clients', *Health & Social Care in the Community*, 18(1): 91-9.

Lewin, G., Vandermeulen, S., and Coster, C. (2006) 'Programs to promote independence at home: how effective are they?', *Journal of the British Society of Gerontology*, 16(3): 24-26.

Lewin, G., Concanen, K., and Youens, D. (2016) 'The Home Independence Program with non-health professionals as care managers: an evaluation', *Clinical Interventions in Aging*, 11: 807-17.

Månsson, M. (2007) *Hemrehabilitering: vad, hur och för vem*, Stockholm: Fortbildning AB/Tidningen Äldreomsorg.

McLeod, B. and Mair, M. (2011) *Evaluation of City of Edinburgh Council Home Care Re-ablement Service*, Edinburgh: Scottish Government Social Research.

Metzelthin, S., Rostgaard, T., Parsons, M., and Burton, E. (2020) 'Development of an internationally accepted definition of reablement: a Delphi study', *Ageing and Society*, 42(3): 703–18.

Ministry of Health (2002) *Health of Older People Strategy*, Wellington: New Zealand Government.

Ministry of Health (2016a) *New Zealand Health Strategy*, Wellington: New Zealand Government.

Ministry of Health (2016b) *Healthy Ageing Strategy*, Wellington: New Zealand Government.

Ministry of Health and Care Services (2012) *Report to the Storting (White Paper) Future Care*, Oslo: Norwegian Government.

Ministry of Social Development Office for Senior Citizens (2001) *New Zealand Positive Ageing Strategy*, Wellington: New Zealand Government.

National Strategy for an Ageing Australia (2001) Commonwealth of Australia, National Strategy for an Ageing Australia [online], Available from: https://ifa.ngo/wp-content/uploads/2012/11/062_Australia-2001-National-Strategy-for-an-Ageing-Australia.pdf

NICE (2018) Intermediate care including reablement: Quality standard [QS173], Manchester: National Institute for Health and Care Excellence.

Northern Ireland Assembly (2011) *Transforming Your Care – A Review of Health and Social Care in Northern Ireland*, Belfast: Northern Ireland Assembly.

NOU 2011 Committee (2011) *Official Norwegian Reports NOU 2011: 11 – Innovation in the Care Services*, Oslo: Ministry of Health and Care Services.

OECD (1994) *Caring for Frail Elderly People: New Directions in Care*, Paris: Organisation for Economic Co-operation and Development.

OECD (2019) *Health at a Glance 2019, OECD Indicators*, Paris: Organisation for Economic Cooperation and Development.

Parker, G., Phelos, K., and Shepperdson, B. (1999) 'Best place of care for older people after acute and during sub-acute illness', Report of a National Survey, Working Paper NHS(WM) 78 05/99.

Parker, G., Bhakta, P., Katbamna, S., Lovett, C., Paisley, S., Parker, S., Phelps, K., Baker, R., Jagger, C., Lindesay, J., Shepperdson, B. and Wilson, A. (2000) 'Best place of care for older people after acute and during subacute illness: a systematic review', *Journal of Health Services Research and Policy*, 5(3): 176–89.

Parsons, C. (2002) 'Showing ideas as causes: The origins of the European Union', *International Organization*, 56(1): 47–84.

Parsons, M., Anderson, C., Senior, H., Chen, X., Kerse, N., Jorgensen, D., Paul, B., Jacobs, S., Stephen, V., and Kilpatrick, J. (2006) *ASPIRE Assessment of Services Promoting Independence and Recovery in Elders*, Auckland: Newzealand Ministry of Health.

Parsons, M., Senior, H., Kerse, N., Chen, M., Jacobs, S., and Anderson, C. (2017) 'Randomised trial of restorative home care for frail older people in New Zealand', *Nursing Older People*, 29(7): 27–33.

Pettersson, C. and Iwarsson, S. (2015) *Vardagsrehabilitering – en kunskapsöversikt*. Förbundet Sveriges Arbetsterapeuter [online], Available from: https://www.arbetsterapeuterna.se/media/1572/vardagsrehabilitering.pdf

Rostad, H.M., Skinner, M.S., Hellesø, R., and Sogstad, M.K.R. (2020) 'Towards specialised and differentiated long-term care services: a cross-sectional study', *BMC Health Services Research*, 20(793): 1–9.

Rostgaard, T. and Graff, L. (2016) *Med hænderne i lommen: Borger og medarbejders samspil og samarbejde i rehabilitering*, Copenhagen: KORA.

Secretary of State for Health (2000) *The NHS Plan: A Plan for Investment, A Plan for Reform*, London: The Stationery Office.

Social Services Act (2014) Lov om ændring af lov om social service, *Lov nr 1524 af 27/12/2014*, Copenhagen: Social- og Indenrigsministeriet, Danske love.

Social Services Improvement Agency (SSIA) (2016) *Reablement Services in Wales: Themed Review of Practice*, Cardiff: SSIA.

Swedish Government Official Report (2017) *SOU 2017:21 Läs mig! National kvalitetsplan för vård och omsorg om äldre personer*.

Thuesen, J., Doh, D., Feiring, M., and Westendorp, R. (2021) 'Reablement and theories of ageing', *Ageing and Society*, 1–13.

Tuntland, H., Aaslund, M.K., Espehaug, B., Førland, O., and Kjeken, I. (2015) 'Reablement in community-dwelling older adults: a randomised controlled trial', *BMC Geriatrics*, 15: 145.

Walker, A. and Maltby, T. (2012) 'Active ageing: a strategic policy solution to demographic ageing in the European Union', *International Journal of Social Welfare*, 21(s1): 117–30.

Weir, A. (2018) 'Effective restorative home support for older people living with dementia and their caregivers: a New Zealand case study', *Cognitive Disorders*, Mthatha: Walter Sisulu University.

WHO (1999) *Active Ageing*, Genéve: World Health Organization.

WHO (2020) *Ageing: Healthy Ageing and Functional Ability*, Genéve: World Health Organization.

4

Reablement as an evolution in home care: a comparison of implementation across five countries

*John Parsons, Elissa Burton, Lea Graff, Silke Metzelthin,
Hilary O'Connell, and Hanne Tuntland*

Introduction

Chapter 2 presents the policy context for reablement across seven countries and highlights the similarity in institutional characteristics across these countries. However, despite this commonality in characteristics and the development of an agreed conceptual understanding of reablement (Metzelthin et al, 2020), there is considerable variation in how reablement is actually implemented across countries. This chapter illustrates the influence of various factors on the implementation of reablement in five countries/regions across the world, namely Denmark, the Netherlands, New Zealand, Norway, and Western Australia (WA) (see more on how ideas of reablement have travelled across the world in Chapter 3 by Feiring et al). The choice of countries is driven by the ability to explore the implementation of reablement up to 2020, with some countries having reablement models that have been in place for over a decade and others being in the situation that reablement was at the stage of small pilots at the time of writing the chapter. The chapter illustrates that the actual implementation of reablement into practice is dependent on contextual factors within the country, and there is a need to consider these factors when introducing and scaling up a multifaceted intervention such as reablement.

A study of implementation offers a systematic approach to explore how to get 'what works' to people who need it with greater speed, fidelity, efficiency, and coverage (Bonell et al, 2012). This chapter utilises constructs and principles from i–PAHRIS (Kitson et al, 2008; Harvey and Kitson, 2015), an established implementation framework, to explore implementation of reablement across the five countries. i-PARIHS is a well validated method of exploring the implementation of initiatives into clinical practice and has four key constructs:

- The innovation construct: relates to the new approach that is being introduced (here, how is reablement defined and delivered as an innovative approach within each country). It also includes the underlying assumption of how the new approach works and what its fit is within the existing systems.

- The recipient construct: considers the impact individuals and teams have in supporting or resisting an innovation (this includes both the perceptions and experience of team members involved in the design and delivery of reablement).
- The context construct: those concerned with the wider environment, both internally (inner context, including leadership and support, culture and organisational priorities) and externally to the organisation (outer context, including policy, social, regulatory and political infrastructures) in which implementation is taking place. This includes the organisational structures for the teams involved in delivering reablement and the policy context within a country or region.
- The facilitation construct: the role of facilitation within implementation of the new approach. This includes those involved in driving and supporting the implementation of reablement. The role of facilitator can operate across the constructs of: innovation (through design and planning); recipient (through change management, team building, and boundary spanning); and context (through political influence/awareness, stakeholder engagement, and networking).

The chapter uses these constructs to explore the implementation of the reablement models across the five countries and the factors that have influenced the implementation of reablement. The different approaches and the challenges and facilitating factors in the implementation are presented and discussed. This adds to a common understanding of the issues around the development and refinement of reablement and acknowledges that, although each of the national health and social care systems have their own unique characteristics, there are common components that need to be addressed to enable successful implementation of reablement.

The innovation construct

In the following section, the innovation construct of the i-PAHRIS framework helps identify how reablement was first delivered and how it may have been considered a new and significantly different intervention, compared to what was otherwise provided. It also considers how reablement required a re-definition of the traditional target group for home care interventions and how the key components within reablement services differed from conventional home care, for instance by being a time-limited intervention with continuous re-assessment (but not in all countries) and for providing training in everyday activities.

Denmark

In Denmark, reablement was initially a bottom-up initiative from the municipality of Fredericia in 2008, aimed at better containing costs and improving quality of life. Similar to conventional home care, reablement services in Denmark are primarily targeted at older people living at home with functional decline, but are only given if the recipient is considered to be motivated, or as it is expressed, 'has the potential'. In contrast to compensatory home care, which is given on a permanent basis, the reablement intervention typically lasts up to 12 weeks (Social- og Indenrigsministeriets Benchmarkingenhed, 2019) and consists of training in daily activities inside and to a lesser degree outside the home, applying a goals-based approach. The client may receive compensatory home care alongside reablement services.

The Netherlands

Reablement is a relatively new approach in Dutch home care, focused on independence, ageing-in-place and cost savings. Chapter 2 by Tuntland et al describes the spread of reablement into a more systemic model across the Netherlands. This chapter instead will focus on the initial implementation at a more local level. Within the Netherlands, reablement was seen as a significant change in service delivery for older people, which required a cultural change. Therefore, there was a strong focus on training of those involved in the delivery of reablement. Between 2014–16, researchers from Maastricht University developed a reablement training programme called 'Stay Active at Home' (Metzelthin et al, 2017). It is a 9-month training, which consists of face-to-face meetings, practical assignments in-between the meetings, and weekly newsletters. The programme aimed to equip home care professionals with the necessary knowledge, skills, self-efficacy, and social support to apply reablement.

Within the small-scale implementation of reablement in the Netherlands, services are implemented alongside usual home care. In contrast to other country approaches, services are not time-limited, and are applicable for all target groups regardless of age who may benefit from review at least once or twice a year to determine whether the service is still required. Personal care and nursing services are provided by small-scale nursing teams. The intensity of the services can vary between a few visits a month to several times a day.

New Zealand

In New Zealand reablement has involved a process of reorientating home care services in response to government policy developed in the early 2000s (Ministry of Health, 2000, 2001), which provided a focus for providers of health services to ensure equitable, timely, affordable, and accessible health services for older people (King et al, 2011; Parsons et al, 2017). It was acknowledged that home care needed to have a rehabilitation and empowerment focus that supported specialist health services for older people. Of relevance to the implementation of reablement is the combined nature of health and social care within New Zealand in relation to both funding and delivery. People with a disability lasting longer than 6 months and aged over 65 years (Māori aged over 55 years) are eligible for reablement services, and as in the Netherlands, reablement services are not time-limited. Finally, services are provided by a private home care organisation contracted by the local health region, and may consist of one visit per day over a 5-day period; however, there are examples where there are up to four visits a day, 7 days per week.

Norway

Local municipalities in Norway were inspired by the successful implementation of reablement in Denmark and started implementing reablement in 2012. The application of reablement was also supported in a national level by the Norwegian Occupational Therapy Association who in 2012 initiated 'Reablement in Norway' (Ness et al, 2012). To date, approximately three out of four Norwegian municipalities are offering reablement services. In common with several countries, the intention behind reablement in Norway was to improve the quality of the home-care services for community-dwelling older adults.

Reablement within Norway is aimed primarily at older adults with a functional decline living in the community and irrespective of diagnosis. Services are often delivered on a daily basis 5 days a week during a reablement period of on average 5 weeks, with a range from 3 to 12 weeks (Langeland et al, 2016).

As is common across the countries, the reablement intervention is based on the meaningful activities the participant has identified as his/her goals. The activity goals deal most frequently with mobility, personal care, and household management (Tuntland et al, 2019). The intervention components are most frequently training in daily activities inside and outside the home, physical exercises to enhance strength, endurance, and balance, home modifications, assistive technology, and adaptations of activity performance (Langeland et al, 2016).

Western Australia

Consideration of the innovation construct within WA illustrates the complexity of the social care landscape and the alignment of reablement within this context. Across Australia, the Commonwealth government has full funding, policy, and operational responsibility for the delivery of aged care services with community-based services being provided through local, state, or nationally based organisations. As described in Chapter 3, reablement arose from a bottom-up initiative to respond to the local context within WA. The first reablement home care programme Home Independence Programme (HIP) was developed in 1999 by Silver Chain, a large and private WA home care provider. The Personal Enablement Programme (PEP) was commenced in 2002 and was like HIP, except participants were referred from hospitals rather than the community. The target group is 65+ (aboriginal and Torres Strait Islander people 50+) with those in need of assistance required to continue living in the community. A successful trial culminated in the WA State Government Home and Community Care Programme (WA HACC) funding Silver Chain to deliver HIP and PEP from 2004 until 2018 and provided an opportunity for a series of research trials of the HIP model. Between 2006 and 2016 the WA HACC undertook a major change of focus from a dependency model of service delivery to an enabling model and the establishment of independent Regional Assessment Services (known as RAS), which separated eligibility and assessment from the provision of care services with a focus on recommendations for appropriate levels of support that build independence and wellbeing (Government of Western Australia Department of Health, 2009; O'Connell, 2013; Government of West Australia Department of Health, 2015).

The recipient construct

This construct of the i-PAHRIS model considers the impact individuals and teams have in supporting or resisting the implementation of reablement. This includes the composition and roles of the reablement team together with the beliefs and values of team members. Overall, it is clear that the implementation of reablement has required a re-orientation of cultural beliefs and assumptions about inter-disciplinary collaboration.

Denmark

Within Denmark, services are delivered by reablement care workers and therapists in cooperation with registered nurses, either organised as a special service unit or integrated into the compensatory home care service unit. Assessment for reablement will often be conducted by a nurse (Bertelsen and Hansen, 2018). The initial delivery of reablement in Denmark was strongly supported by the Association of Occupational Therapists (see also Chapter 3 by Feiring et al).

Being mandatory by law since 2015, reablement seems to fit well into existing practises in the Danish municipalities, where help-to-self-help had been a guiding principle for decades, though not with the same impact as the much more focused reablement approach (Petersen et al, 2017). However, integrating the reablement perspective in regular home care services has proven difficult because of existing and strong values of performing services in a more traditional way, meaning doing things *for* instead of *with* the participant, but also because of organisational factors, such as lack of time and resources (Rostgaard and Graff, 2016; Bertelsen and Hansen, 2018).

Danish studies show that implementing reablement can be both challenging and rewarding for home care/reablement care workers (see also Chapter 9 by Rostgaard and Graff). It is demanding in its focus on producing self-efficacy, but also provides opportunities for skill learning and inter-disciplinary collaboration (Petersen and Kjellberg, 2016). For therapists, reablement fits well within their existing practice and professional paradigm. Integrating nurses in the reablement interventions has proven somewhat difficult, with many evaluations showing a low degree of fit with both the nurses' existing practice and their values. Integrating nurses in reablement thus requires attention to their distinct work tasks and the organisation of these (Rostgaard and Graff, 2016).

The Netherlands

In the Netherlands, reablement is strongly guided by the nursing discipline. Each reablement team is guided by a district nurse, who coordinates the team and is also responsible for assessing participants' needs and creating and evaluating the support plan. The other team members are nurses or nurse assistants where the latter provide most of the personal care (such as assistance with washing and dressing). Domestic support is provided by reablement care workers, who work individually under supervision of a manager. Most services are provided once a week for approximately 2–3 hours.

Within the Netherlands, the 'Stay Active at Home' programme is based on the assumption that staff training is a key element for the implementation of reablement, as it asks for behavioural change in nurses and reablement care workers, who have to change their day-to-day professional behaviour, before a behavioural change in participants can be reached (Metzelthin et al, 2017). The evidence for the impact of the recipient level construct is limited to date within the Netherlands. However, the focus on training is seen as a key strategy for implementation of reablement to support and manage the views, knowledge, and beliefs of those involved in delivering reablement services.

New Zealand

In common with the Netherlands, a key focus in New Zealand has related to the training needs of providers of reablement services (home care nurses, therapists, and reablement care workers, with the attainment of the participant's own goals highlighted). In addition, there needed to be a reorientation of the focus of the home care team from primarily treating disease and 'taking care' of participants, to maximising function and comfort and working as an integrated inter-professional team with shared goals. Finally, there needed to be comprehensive assessment and diagnosis leading to the development of a multifaceted treatment plan that includes various combinations of exercise, behavioural changes, environmental adjustments and adaptive equipment, counselling and support, and training and education of the older person, family, and friends (Parsons et al, 2015).

Reablement services in New Zealand have separate needs assessment and provider functions. As a result of the need for a comprehensive assessment, the inter-RAI home care and contact assessments were adopted and slowly integrated as the tool used by the needs assessors.

Within New Zealand, integration of reablement into the practice of clinicians working as coordinators in home care has been challenging and, in most cases, this has aligned to individual discipline's areas of expertise. The model has often been viewed by home care coordinator staff as more complex than traditional home care delivery. In addition to the funding system, the enhanced supervision required by the coordinator of the unregulated support workers, the increased requirement for liaison with primary and secondary care, and the need to develop skills around goal setting and planning have all been seen as adding complexity to the provision of home care. This has often led to issues relating to a perception of an increased workload but with data showing that there is also increased job satisfaction and a reduction in staff turnover (King et al, 2012; Jacobs et al, 2018).

Norway

Staff delivering reablement in Norway are primarily physiotherapists, occupational therapists, nurses, and reablement care workers, with an average of four different professions in the team (Langeland et al, 2016). The therapists supervise the reablement care workers in how to encourage and assist the older person in the daily training. Therapy personnel are often the ones who perform the needs assessment and assessment of the effects of the intervention with an inherent focus on rehabilitation principles.

Furthermore, the experience in Norway has shown that when implementing reablement, the team faces several barriers. The establishment of reablement is a complex process that takes place both within the service, and at the organisational and societal levels. From the healthcare worker's perspective, establishing reablement involves more than replicating a service model from elsewhere and mechanically learning new methods. It involves developing old practices into new practices, and requires a service tailored to local conditions (Moe and Brinchmann, 2018).

Facilitating factors for the development of reablement teams include a focus on inter-disciplinarity, professional autonomy and flexibility, and working towards common goals (Moe et al, 2017). Moreover, on a structural level, having meeting places, sufficient time to apply professional knowledge when supporting older adults in everyday activities, and an improved framework for cooperation, are seen as facilitating factors (Hjelle et al, 2018; Vik, 2018). Barriers include varying morale of the professionals, care culture versus rehabilitation culture, the varying status of professionals, and expectations of economic savings (Moe et al, 2017).

Western Australia

RAS reablement services in WA are delivered by an RAS assessor within the assessment process, with referral to a home care provider to deliver the service. From 2011, people receiving reablement were assessed for eligibility by RAS staff as part of the WA HACC Programme and referred through to the reablement care manager, namely physiotherapist, occupational therapist, or registered nurse), who determined a structured programme to assist the person to reach their goals. The assessment staff determine whether an older person requires support through the CHSP and recommends the support required. This system has been through considerable changes over the last two decades in terms of structure and responsibilities of different roles involved in assessment and delivery of reablement services.

The context construct

This refers to how the inner and outer context may facilitate implementation. The inner context includes the local and organisational setting of the reablement team and its embeddedness, and which illustrates the differences and similarities across the countries. Outer context refers to the wider social care and health system in which the organisation is based, and reflects the policy, social, regulatory, and political infrastructures surrounding the local context, not least the funding arrangement. The outer context considers issues that interact with the content presented in Chapter 2.

Denmark

In Denmark, at a national level, the implementation of reablement has been supported throughout by the main trade unions, and perhaps most importantly, by both legislation, and financially by large funding schemes from the National Health Board. The government has been active in helping the municipalities implement reablement by funding training courses via the relevant national boards. Studies on evidence- and practice-based knowledge of reablement were completed in 2012–13 to aid in developing an official handbook of reablement by the National Health Board (Sundhedsstyrelsen, 2016). The studies were also used by the Board to develop an evidence-based model of the organisation of reablement, which was tested in two municipalities and evaluated thoroughly (Lauritzen et al, 2017). Likewise, the national legislation on reablement from 2015 was followed up by a nationwide study of reablement practice (Rambøll Management Consulting, 2017). The implementation has also been supported by adding reablement to the curriculum in the home care/support workers educations.

Municipalities can, but are not obliged to, let private for-profit providers of home care participate in delivering reablement. Danish studies report contradicting opinions on whether the private providers have the financial incentive to deliver reablement (Bertelsen and Hansen, 2018) although it is under-researched (Petersen et al, 2017).

When funding reablement, municipalities may choose an activity-based funding model related to the participant's functional level and complexity of the intervention. Some municipalities are experimenting with combining this funding model with a result-based model to provide the private for-profit providers with incentives to work towards maximum independence for the participant. The vast majority of reablement provision, however, is publicly provided (Rambøll Management Consulting, 2016).

In addition, the length of time since the initial set-up of reablement, locally from 2007 and in legislation from 2017, and the integration of reablement into standard practice to support older people, has impacted on the policy, social, regulatory, and political infrastructures in Denmark, in such a way that the philosophy of reablement is now strongly institutionalised.

The Netherlands

In the Netherlands, important contextual factors both hinder and assist the implementation of the reablement approach. It is recognised that the core components of training and interdisciplinarity, identified in the previous section, are key to the potential spread of reablement within the Netherlands. In addition, there is an acknowledgement that the current fee-for-service funding model creates perverse incentives to stimulate the quantity of care rather than the quality of care: the more services are delivered, the more money home care providers will earn. Therefore, there is an acknowledged need for a new sustainable funding model that facilitates goal-oriented, holistic, and person-centred home care that takes into account the capabilities and resources of participants instead of focusing on disease and dependency (Elissen, 2017; van den Bulck et al, 2019). Considerable effort is presently being placed on the development of a new funding model as reablement is scaled up within the country. As a result, in 2017, on behalf of the Dutch

Ministry of Health, Welfare and Sport, the Dutch Healthcare Authority initiated a joint venture with three Dutch universities to create a knowledge base for the development of a new funding model for home care in the Netherlands. Rather than incentivising the volume of care, the new model should incentivise home care professionals to – based on their professional knowledge and experience – provide high-quality care that is tailored to participants' needs (van den Bulck et al, 2019).

Furthermore, it is assumed that a strong and shared vision regarding the new way of delivering home care delivery is needed, including supporting organisational procedures and policies (Metzelthin et al, 2017). Within the 'Stay Active at Home' programme, all staff across organisations were regularly informed about the aims, content, and progress of the training.

New Zealand

A mixture of for-profit and not-for-profit private organisations are contracted to deliver home care in New Zealand. An increasing number of these are large national providers, whereas there remains a small number who only provide services within one or two health regions. The ability of smaller organisations to effectively implement reablement has been variable, whereas in several cases the learning within larger organisations allows for the transfer of experience from previous health regions where they may have been involved in the delivery of the restorative model.

There has been an emphasis on modifying the model of funding to incentivise providers to apply the principles of the model. A case-mix funding model was developed and implemented that uses the inter-RAI contact (older people with non-complex needs) and home care assessments (for complex needs) (Parsons et al, 2018). Casemix classification is a systematic approach to quantifying the relationship between patient-driven variables and resource use. It places healthcare cases into groups where members of the group are clinically similar, and use similar amounts of care. Achieving this grouping consistently allows the alignment of best evidence interventions to members of each group and appropriate targeting of interventions (Parsons et al, 2018). Within New Zealand this has been key to incentivising home care providers to align service provision to the principles of reablement.

Norway

Funding of reablement in Norway is on a fee-for-service basis with separate compensation on a service level for both physiotherapy and general practitioner input (Bersvendsen, 2020). The local implementation of reablement was from an early stage supported economically by the Norwegian Ministry of Health and Care Services through different stimulation funds. Since then, the government has supported the implementation of reablement in several white papers and other governmental plans (Meld, 2015, Norwegian Ministry of Health and Care Services, 2015). Moreover, the government-commissioned implementation was followed by research documenting the effects and impacts of reablement (Langeland et al, 2016; Langeland et al, 2019).

Western Australia

There is considerable complexity when considering the context construct within Australia. The aged care sector in Australia has been undergoing major reform for some years and home care is moving towards a more consumer-driven, market-based system. While WA has been on the 'reablement journey' for some years, the Commonwealth government has only more recently committed to reablement being part of the future of home and community care in Australia, with the adoption and mandating of wellness and reablement in contracts and through resources available to RAS and home care providers. There are, however, still systematic barriers to the adoption and delivery of reablement approaches within all the states and territories of Australia. The success of reablement is, for example, severely hampered by the current task and volume environment that CHSP programme providers operate within, which rewards increasing levels of support and not decreasing levels. Second, a philosophy within the sector of older people being provided *to* rather than partnered *with* over a long period of time has resulted in older people and their carers/families not necessarily seeing the value in, or they are reluctant to engage with, reablement and have an expectation of traditional services being provided.

The facilitation context

Facilitation is the process of a person or persons making the implementation of an intervention into practice easier for those performing the intervention (Harvey & Kitson, 2015). This is in recognition that relying on practitioners to change their practice to a required standard autonomously is often less successful when compared to a facilitated change in practice. Facilitation appears to be a key feature across the five countries considered in this chapter, but with a different emphasis placed on the fulfilment of this role (see also Chapter 3 by Feiring et al for an analysis of entrepreneurs and driving forces).

Denmark

Being a bottom-up initiative, the municipality of Fredericia has been the foremost facilitator of reablement in Denmark, and the municipalities themselves have been the most important facilitators. Other important facilitators are the National Board of Social Services, who was the responsible agency until 2015, and the National Health Board since then. Also, the continued support from influential trade unions representing social care workers and occupational therapists, and from the large organisation representing older people and their relatives, Dan Age, seems very important.

New Zealand

A major factor in successful implementation in New Zealand has been the facilitator role played by the Funding and Planning portfolio manager within a health region (who is responsible for strategic responses for the health needs of the population at a regional level), and the local manager of the assessment agency. To a certain extent, the managers of the homecare agencies have also been the facilitators (Senior et al, 2014; Jacobs et al, 2018).

Norway

In Norway, the Norwegian Occupational Therapy Association promoted reablement extensively to national and local health authorities, as well as to interested clinicians, administrators and scholars nationwide. The association created a widespread enthusiasm for reablement, encouraging and supporting clinicians and municipalities that wanted to start implementing the new service.

The Netherlands

The researchers from Maastricht University developed the 'Stay Active at Home' programme in co-creation with relevant Dutch stakeholders (nurses and other healthcare professionals, older adults, policy makers, training officers, managers, and the board of directors) (Metzelthin et al, 2017). By participating in the development process, they became enthusiastic about the programme and felt responsible for spreading the programme inside and outside their organisation. Also, the stepwise implementation approach, namely conducting a pilot study, an exploratory trial before a cluster randomised controlled trial started, facilitated the implementation of the programme, as relevant experiences could be made that were used to further improve the feasibility and (cost-)effectiveness of the programme (Metzelthin et al, 2017). Finally, as addressed earlier, the support from the inner and outer context is/was important to facilitate the implementation of reablement.

Western Australia

The development of the Home Independence Programme (HIP) in 1999 by Silver Chain, a large West Australian home care provider, seems to have been the enabling force behind reablement being introduced across Australia. A major factor in the successful implementation of both HIP, PEP, and subsequently the RAS wellness approach, was the role played by the WA State Government Home and Community Care Programme (WA HACC), who funded Silver Chain's independence programmes, adopted wellness as the underpinning philosophy for all service delivery in WA, and introduced the RAS who would assess the need for home care services through the lens of wellness and reablement.

Reablement in WA commenced and was driven through the introduction of HIP and PEP and subsequent 'Independence Programs' developed by one health and community care organisation. The WA state government Aged Care Policy Directorate played a key facilitator role through strategic support and ongoing funding. As the Australian homecare landscape changes, reablement is now an underpinning philosophy of the Aged Care reform agenda, and therefore predominantly funded by the Commonwealth Government, who may, along with the Regional Assessment Services, be viewed as fulfilling the role of facilitator of reablement in Australia.

Discussion

This chapter has presented a number of factors to be considered in the implementation of reablement. To successfully implement a new policy and practice approach, it is not sufficient to determine that a model in another geographical area is effective (Harrison and Grantham, 2018). Transferring reablement models from one region/country to another requires an understanding of how reablement is organised differently across multiple jurisdictions and how differences in organisational set-ups and cultures affect the transfer of ideas and innovations both within and across geographical contexts (Gray et al, 2017). As shown in the chapter, the implementation of reablement across the five countries/regions has several common features, in addition to features that are unique to each area. In the following, we will highlight these, and also point at some additional features which seem to have been influential.

Common features across the five countries/regions

The description of reablement within the innovation construct shows that there are key common features in the composition of reablement across the five countries/regions, and which sets the approach apart from what has previously been provided. They all share a focus on community-dwelling older adults with functional decline, and are aligned with the underlying theory that integrates knowledge and evidence from a wide range of rehabilitation, social, learning, and behaviour change theories. A further common feature is at the recipient construct level, where an interdisciplinary approach that focuses on changing the philosophy from one, where delivery of care may create dependency, to the provision of care, which maximises independence and health-related quality of life and reduces care needs (Moe and Gårseth-Nesbakk, 2015; Tuntland, 2017).

The differences in the focus for implementing reablement may predominantly be due to the variation at the level of the context construct across the countries. For example, the degree of integration of reablement services within home care shows considerable variation. In New Zealand, there is full integration, whereas in Norway there was a focus on the integration of rehabilitation and home care resources. In Denmark, there is a split model with most municipalities delivering reablement using home care staff and others using designated reablement teams consisting of therapists and/or reablement care workers in cooperation with regular home care staff.

Each country would appear to have had success in the refinement of different aspects of reablement service provision across the i-PAHRIS constructs. In New Zealand, there has been a strong focus on comprehensive geriatric assessment using inter-RAI and the development of funding models to provide incentives to contracted organisations in line with economic theory (Bisceglia et al, 2018; Kazungu et al, 2018). In Denmark, considerable innovation has occurred in education and resourcing, with a demonstrable impact on service quality (Sundhedsstyrelsen, 2016). Norway has concentrated significant effort into developing a strong therapy focus with occupational therapy championing reablement services (Ness et al, 2012). Australia has demonstrated unique approaches to assessment and resourcing of staff within reablement service provision. The Netherlands has been able to choose features from the different models of reablement implemented in other countries.

Goal-setting

There is conflicting evidence relating to the ability to set meaningful participant-centred goals within reablement with Danish evidence that goals are often constrained by available services (Kjellberg et al, 2012; Rostgaard and Graff, 2016). This is supported by research exploring goal-setting within rehabilitation settings where goals aligned to clinician priorities is a common issue (Levack et al, 2011; Parsons et al, 2016), with such 'privileged goals' representing known territory for clinicians as they relate to activities that they were comfortable performing and addressed their main work responsibilities and priorities. However, in New Zealand and Norway, training for clinicians in the use of specific goal-setting tools resulted in a greater emphasis on participant-driven goals (Parsons et al, 2012; Moe et al, 2017; Tuntland et al, 2019). The level of engagement of participants within reablement service provision is closely linked to evidence highlighting the impact of participatory goal-setting (Levack et al, 2006; Rosewilliam et al, 2011). In addition, demonstrable alignment of the values of service with those of the participant and their family (Wong-Cornall et al, 2017), a focus on enhancing motivation (Lauritzen et al, 2017; Petersen et al, 2017; Bertelsen and Hansen, 2018), and involvement of the family (Hjelle et al, 2017; Wong-Cornall et al, 2017), were also associated with effective engagement of the participant within the reablement process.

Teamwork

The focus on integrated and interdisciplinary teamwork across reablement teams appears to be a significant factor in delivering these changes in key outcomes. However, there is also evidence that the team approach led to higher levels of staff satisfaction (Hjelle et al, 2016; Bertelsen and Hansen, 2018; Eliassen et al, 2018) and reduced staff turnover (King et al, 2012). It is interesting to note that this increased satisfaction is accompanied by evidence that staff finds the implementation of reablement to be challenging because of organisational factors (such as lack of time) and motivational factors (such as reablement care workers preferring to work in a more traditional compensatory manner) (Cochrane et al, 2016).

Staff training

A common feature is the acknowledgement of the need for robust training to enable any necessary change in the culture of dependency among home care or community health and social care workers and to manage the complex nature of the participants. There is evidence from a number of countries that the implementation of the model is challenging for health professionals and may involve delegation of some tasks, that may have been aligned to specific disciplines, or to the reablement care workers (Parsons et al, 2015). Conversely, there is a level of divergence in the disciplines involved in the delivery of reablement services. In New Zealand, the model primarily uses registered nurses to undertake assessments and coordinate services with reablement care workers providing assistance and support to the participant. Therapy input is provided in a consulting or advisory capacity (Parsons et al, 2015). This is a model that has been replicated in the Netherlands with registered nurses being the key discipline involved in coordination of reablement. Within Denmark and Norway, the delivery of reablement is most often led by therapists in cooperation with reablement care workers, with registered nurses having either a minor or unclear role. In the WA model, initially reablement was delivered by therapists and nurses with assistance from support staff. However, more recently there has been innovation around the use of non-health professionals in assessment and coordination roles.

Organisational composition for reablement service delivery

There is considerable variation in the composition of organisations providing reablement services. In Norway and Denmark, staff are employed directly by the municipality. In Denmark, there are a few examples of private for-profit providers of home care offering reablement services under contract with the municipalities, whereas most providers in the other countries are contracted organisations that are a mix of for-profit and not-for-profit non-governmental organisations. However, in general, there is evidence to suggest that the type of organisation (for-profit versus not-for-profit) has little effect on the participant or staff satisfaction (Schmid, 2002) and that inter-organisational relationships and communication is a far more important factors in effective service provision (Powell Davies et al, 2008; Eklund and Wilhelmson, 2009).

Facilitation

Facilitation is seen as a key component to successful implementation (Harvey and Kitson, 2015). Across the five countries, there were various approaches to the facilitation of implementation. Within New Zealand and Denmark, this was undertaken by regional and local managers in the health region or municipality. In Norway, the national occupational therapy association played a key advocacy and facilitation role. Within Australia, the Silver Chain organisation and state and Commonwealth governments were key to facilitating implementation. An important issue to consider here is that of professional power and the role that this may play in the degree of success of a new innovation such as reablement. Ferlie et al (2005) illustrate the role that health professions can play to either increase or retard the spread of innovations. An example of this in the case of reablement is the significant role played by the Norwegian Occupational Therapy Association in the scaling up of reablement. Or in the case of Denmark, the importance of the support from an interest organisation like Dan Age with a membership count representing one in five of the total population.

Consideration of the other factors that impacted on the implementation of reablement across the five countries/regions illustrates the importance of a coordinated approach to engaging with staff and older people around the model. The importance of engaging with staff and acknowledging the complex nature of this engagement has been shown to be crucial for the successful implementation of interventions within healthcare (Moore et al, 2014).

Spread of reablement across the five countries/regions

Within New Zealand, reablement type services have been implemented across the majority of semi-autonomous health regions. In Denmark, all municipalities have implemented reablement, driven by legislation. In a similar fashion, Norway has seen reablement implemented across three out of four municipalities. The Norwegian model is a well-developed approach to scaling up and spread of reablement into a new municipality. In contrast, the complex nature of the health system in Australia with both federal and state funding and policy has meant that the spread of reablement has been variable and at times lost in translation. In the states of WA and Victoria, a reablement approach became the underpinning philosophy of both states with regards to how support was provided to people receiving home and community care services (Victorian Department of Human Services, 2008; O'Connell, 2013). Although not universally adopted, several service providers across Australia have changed the way their services are delivered and have developed reablement-focused support services and programmes. In the Netherlands, reablement is in its infancy with small pilot projects informing robust research to build the evidence base within the local context. It is proposed that a major factor in driving the scale and spread in New Zealand, Denmark, and Norway, is the centralised policy and planning structures within these fairly small countries, which has enabled a coherent and sustained approach to widespread implementation.

Scaling up complex health and social care interventions to large populations is not a straightforward task. The scale-up of such interventions addresses the system/infrastructure issues that arise during full-scale implementation (Nelson et al, 2002). Without intentional, guided efforts to scale up, it can take many years for a new evidence-based intervention to be broadly implemented. For the past decade, models of scale-up have been proposed that move beyond earlier paradigms that assumed ideas and practices would successfully spread through a combination of publication, policy, training, and example (Shaw et al, 2017). It is now accepted that funding pilot and research projects to develop and implement reablement on a small scale, a common feature presented in this chapter, is not enough to ensure that the model developed and refined in the pilot/research can be implemented elsewhere.

Conclusion

Implementation of an intervention like reablement is a complex and dynamic process influenced by many factors. Translating innovative models requires an understanding of the attributes of each model, the context in which it was developed, and the context into which the successful model will be spread. It is also imperative to have a clear formulation of how to adapt and adopt the model in the new context. Transferring models from one jurisdiction to another requires an understanding of how reablement is organised differently across multiple jurisdictions and how differences in organisations affect the translatability of ideas and innovations both within and across jurisdictions. Moreover, it is important to understand how the effects of policy, financing, and regulation constrain or encourage organisation and activities among providers to deliver care, and how these impact outcomes for the older person and family/caregiver.

This chapter has shown factors that have influenced the variation in the implementation of reablement across five countries. Despite variations in health and social care systems across the countries, the driving forces are similar, namely the sustainability threats due to the demographic change, lack of qualified personnel, and demand for home care service exceeding supply. Implementation of reablement across five countries has several common features, as well as features unique to each country, and this highlights the importance of context in the successful implementation of complex interventions.

References

Bersvendsen, T. (2020) *Effects of home-based reablement: a micro-econometric approach*, Oslo: University of Agder School of Business and Law.

Bertelsen, A.T.M. and Hansen, M.B. (2018) *Hverdagsrehabilitering og velfærdsinnovation i ældreplejens organisering [Reablement − specialised or integrated?]*, Ålborg: Ålborg University.

Bisceglia, M., Cellini, R., and Grilli, L. (2018) 'Regional regulators in health care service under quality competition: a game theoretical model', *Journal of Health Economics*, 27(11): 1821–42.

Bonell, C., Fletcher, A., Morton, M., Lorenc, T., and Moore, L. (2012) 'Realist randomised controlled trials: a new approach to evaluating complex public health interventions', *Social Science & Medicine*, 75(12): 2299–306.

Cochrane, A., Furlong, M., McGilloway, S., Molloy, D.W., Stevenson, M., and Donnelly, M. (2016) 'Time-limited home–care reablement services for maintaining and improving the functional independence of older adults', *Cochrane Database of Systematic Reviews*, 10: CD010825.

Eklund, K. and Wilhelmson, K. (2009) 'Outcomes of coordinated and integrated interventions targeting frail elderly people: a systematic review of randomised controlled trials', *Health & Social Care in the Community*, 17(5): 447–58.

Eliassen, M., Henriksen, N.O., and Moe, S. (2018) 'Physiotherapy supervision of home trainers in interprofessional reablement teams', *Journal of Interprofessional Care*, 33(5): 512–18.

Elissen, A., Metzelthin, S., van den Bulck, A., Verbeek, H., and Ruwaard, D. (2017) *Case-mix classificatie als basis voor bekostiging van wijkverpleging. Een verkennend onderzoek in opdracht van Meander Groep Zuid-Limburg*, Maastricht, the Netherlands: Maastricht University.

Ferlie, E., Fitzgerald, L., Wood, M., and Hawkins, C. (2005) 'The nonspread of innovations: the mediating role of professionals', *Academy of Management Journal*, 48(1): 117–34.

Government of Western Australia Department of Health (2009) *Western Australian (WA) Home and Community Care (HACC) Program Assessment Framework Service Redesign*, Perth: Government of Western Australia Department of Health.

Government of West Australia Department of Health (2015) *Western Australia Assessment Framework: A Journey*, Perth, WA: Government of West Australia Department of Health.

Greenhalgh, T., Wherton, J., Papoutsi, C., Lynch, J., Hughes, G., A'Court, C., Hinder, S., Fahy, N., Procter, R., and Shaw, S. (2017) 'Beyond adoption: a new framework for theorizing and evaluating nonadoption, abandonment, and challenges to the scale-up, spread, and sustainability of health and care technologies', *Journal of Medical Internet Research*, 19(11): e367.

Harrison, M.I. and Grantham, S. (2018) 'Learning from implementation setbacks: identifying and responding to contextual challenges', *Learning Health Systems*, e10068.

Harvey, G. and Kitson, A. (2015) 'PARIHS revisited: from heuristic to integrated framework for the successful implementation of knowledge into practice', *Implementation Science*, 11(1): 33.

Hjelle, K.M., Tuntland, H., Førland, O., and Alvsvåg, H. (2016) 'Driving-forces for home-based reablement: a qualitative study of older adults' experiences', *Health & Social Care in the Community*, 25(5): 1581–9.

Hjelle, K.M., Tuntland, H., Førland, O., and Alvsvåg, H. (2017) 'Driving forces for home-based reablement: a qualitative study of older adults' experiences', *Health & Social Care in the Community*, 25(5): 1581–9.

Hjelle, K.M., Skutle, O., Alvsvåg, H., and Førland, O. (2018) 'Reablement teams' roles: a qualitative study of interdisciplinary teams' experiences', *Journal of Multidisciplinary Healthcare*, 11: 305.

Jacobs, S.P., Parsons, M., Rouse, P., Parsons, J., and Gunderson-Reid, M. (2018) 'Using benchmarking to assist the improvement of service quality in home support services for older people – IN TOUCH (Integrated Networks Towards Optimising Understanding of Community Health)', *Evaluation and Program Planning*, 67: 113–21.

Kazungu, J.S., Barasa, E.W., Obadha, M., and Chuma, J. (2018) 'What characteristics of provider payment mechanisms influence health care providers' behaviour? A literature review', *The International Journal of Health Planning Management*, 33(4): e892–905.

King, A.I.I., Parsons, M., Robinson, E., and Jørgensen, D. (2011) 'Assessing the impact of a restorative home care service in New Zealand: a cluster randomised controlled trial', *Health & Social Care in the Community*, 20(4): 365–74.

King, A.I.I., Parsons, M., and Robinson, E. (2012) 'A restorative home care intervention in New Zealand: perceptions of paid caregivers', *Health & Social Care in the Community*, 20(1): 70–9.

Kitson, A.L., Rycroft-Malone, J., Harvey, G., McCormack, B., Seers, K., and Titchen, A. (2008) 'Evaluating the successful implementation of evidence into practice using the PARiHS framework: theoretical and practical challenges', *Implementation Science*, 3: 1.

Kjellberg, P., Hauge-Helgestad, A., Madsen, M.H., and Rasmussen, S.R. (2013) *Kortlægning af kommunernes erfaringer med rehabilitering pa ældreområdet*, Odense: Socialstyrelsen.

Langeland, E., Førland, O., Aas, E., Birkeland, A., Folkestad, B., Kjeken, I., Jacobsen, F.F., and Tuntland, H. (2016) *Modeller for hverdagsrehabilitering – en følgeevaluering i norske kommuner. Effekter for brukerne og gevinster for kommunene?*, Bergen: Senter for omsorgsforskning vest: Høgskolen i Bergen, CHARM.

Langeland, E., Tuntland, H., Folkestad, B., Førland, O., Jacobsen, F., and Kjeken, I. (2019) 'A multicenter investigation of reablement in Norway: a clinical controlled trial', *BMC Geriatrics*, 19(29).

Lauritzen, H.H., Bjerre, M., Graff, L., Rostgaard, T., Casier, F., and Fridberg, T. (2017) *Rehabilitering på ældreområdet: Afprøvning af en model for rehabiliteringsforløb i to kommuner [Test of a Rehabilitation Programme Model in Two Municipalities]*, Copenhagen: Sfi – Det Nationale Forskningscenter For Velfærd.

Levack, W.M., Taylor, K., Siegert, R.J., Dean, S.G., McPherson, K.M., and Weatherall, M. (2006) 'Is goal planning in rehabilitation effective? A systematic review', *Clinical Rehabilitation*, 20(9): 739.

Levack, W.M., Dean, S.G., Siegert, R.J., and McPherson, K.M. (2011) 'Navigating patient-centered goal setting in inpatient stroke rehabilitation: how clinicians control the process to meet perceived professional responsibilities', *Patient Education and Counseling*, 85(2): 206–13.

Meld, St. (2015) *Report to the Storting (White Paper) Summary: The Primary Health and Care Services of Tomorrow – Localised and Integrated*, Oslo: Norwegian Ministry of Health and Care Services.

Metzelthin, S., Zijlstra, G.A., Van Rossum, E., de Man-van Ginkel, J.M., Resnick, B., Lewin, G., Parsons, M., and Kempen, G.I. (2017) '"Doing with …" rather than "doing for …" older adults: rationale and content of the "Stay Active at Home" programme', *Clinical Rehabilitation*, 31(11): 1419–30.

Metzelthin, S., Rostgaard, T., Parsons, M., and Burton, E. (2020) 'Development of an internationally accepted definition of reablement: a Delphi study', *Ageing and Society*, 42(3): 703–18.

Ministry of Health (2000) *New Zealand Health Care Strategy*, Wellington, New Zealand: Ministry of Health.

Ministry of Health (2001) *The Primary Health Care Strategy*, Wellington, New Zealand: Ministry of Health.

Moe, A., Ingstad, K., and Brataas, H.V. (2017) 'Patient influence in home-based reablement for older persons: qualitative research', *BMC Health Services Research*, 17(1): 736.

Moe, C. and Brinchmann, B. (2018) 'Tailoring reablement: a grounded theory study of establishing reablement in a community setting in Norway', *Health & Social Care in the Community*, 26(1): 113–21.

Moe, C. and Gårseth-Nesbakk, L. (2015) 'Hverdagsrehabilitering som innovasjon. Økt oppmerksomhet om aktørers samspill [Reablement as Innovation: Increased Attention Regarding Collaboration]', in O.J. Andersen, L. Gårseth- Nesbakk and T. Bondas (eds) *Innovasjoner i offentlig tjenesteyting [Innovations in Public Service Delivery]*, Bergen: Fagbokforlaget, 87–105

Moore, G., Audrey, S., Barker, M., Bond, L., Bonell, C., Hardeman, W., Moore, L., O'Cathain, A., Tinati, T., and Wight, D. (2014) 'Process evaluation of complex interventions', *BMJ*, 350 1–133.

Nelson, E.C., Batalden, P.B., Huber, T.P., Mohr, J.J., Godfrey, M.M., Headrick, L.A., and Wasson, J.H. (2002) 'Microsystems in health care: Part 1. Learning from high-performing front-line clinical units', *The Joint Commission Journal on Quality Improvement*, 28(9): 472–93.

Ness, N., Laberg, T., Haneborg, M., Granbo, R., Færevaag, L., and Butli, H. (2012) *Hverdagsmestring og hverdagsrehabilitering*, Samarbeid mellom Norsk Ergoterapeutforbund, Norsk Fysioterapeutforbund og Norsk Sykepleierforbund.

Norwegian Ministry of Health and Care Services (2015) *Care Plan 2020: The Government's Plan for the Care Services Field for 2015–2020*, Oslo: Ministry of Health and Care Services.

O'Connell, H. (2013) *Challenging Community Care with Wellness: An Implementation Overview of the WA HACC Program's Wellness Approach*, Western Australia: Community West inc.

Parsons, J., Rouse, P., Robinson, E.M., Sheridan, N., and Connolly, M.J. (2012) 'Goal setting as a feature of homecare services for older people: does it make a difference?', *Age and Ageing*, 41(1): 24–9.

Parsons, J., Mathieson, S., and Parsons, M. (2015) 'Home care: an opportunity for physiotherapy', *New Zealand Journal of Physiotherapy*, 43(1): 24–31.

Parsons, J., Plant, S.E., Slark, J., Tyson, S.F. (2016) 'How active are patients in setting goals during rehabilitation after stroke? A qualitative study of clinician perceptions', *Disability and Rehabilitation*, 40(3): 309–16.

Parsons, M., Senior, H., Kerse, N., Chen, M., Jacobs, S., and Anderson, C. (2017) 'Randomised trial of restorative home care for frail older people in New Zealand', *Nursing Older People*, 29(7): 27–33.

Parsons, M., Rouse, P., Sajtos, L., Harrison, J., Parsons, J., and Gestro, L. (2018) 'Developing and utilising a new funding model for home-care services in New Zealand', *Health & Social Care in the Community*, 26(3): 345–55.

Petersen, A. and Kjellberg, P.K. (2016) *Det gode hverdagsliv i Egedal kommune*, Copenhagen: KORA.

Petersen, A., Graff, L., Rostgaard, T., Kjellberg, J., and Kjellberg, P. (2017) *Rehabilitering på ældreomradet. Hvad fortæller danske undersøgelser os om kommunernes arbejde med rehabilitering i hjemmeplejen?*, Copenhagen: Sundhedsstyrelsen.

Powell Davies, G., Williams, A.M., Larsen, K., Perkins, D., Roland, M., and Harris, M.F. (2008) 'Coordinating primary health care: an analysis of the outcomes of a systematic review', *Medical Journal of Australia*, 188: S65–8.

Rambøll Management Consulting (2016) *Innovationspartnerskaber om Rehabilitering*, København: Rambøll Management Consulting.

Rambøll Management Consulting (2017) *Praksisundersøgelse af Servicelovens § 83a*, Copenhagen: Rambøll.

Rosewilliam, S., Roskell, C.A., and Pandyan, A.D. (2011) 'A systematic review and synthesis of the quantitative and qualitative evidence behind patient-centred goal setting in stroke rehabilitation', *Clinical Rehabilitation*, 25(6): 501.

Rostgaard, T. and Graff, L. (2016) *Med hænderne i lommen. Borger og medarbejders samspil og samarbejde i rehabilitering*, Copenhagen: KORA.

Schmid, H. (2002) 'Relationships between organizational properties and organizational effectiveness in three types of nonprofit human service organizations', *Public Personnel Management*, 31(3): 377–96.

Senior, H.E., Parsons, M., Kerse, N., Chen, M.-H., Jacobs, S., Hoorn, S.V., and Anderson, C.S. (2014) 'Promoting independence in frail older people: a randomised controlled trial of a restorative care service in New Zealand', *Age and Ageing*, 43(3): 418–24.

Shaw, J., Shaw, S., Wherton, J., Hughes, G., and Greenhalgh, T. (2017) 'Studying scale-up and spread as social practice: theoretical introduction and empirical case study', *Journal of Medical Internet Research*, 19(7): e244.

Social- og Indenrigsministeriets Benchmarkingenhed (2019) *Rehabilitering på ældreomradet efter § 83a i Serviceloven [Reablement in elder care inder §83a in Social Services Act]*, Copenhagen: Social- og Indenrigsministeriets Benchmarkingenhed.

Sundhedsstyrelsen (2016) *Håndbog i rehabiliteringsforløb på ældreområdet. [Handbook on reablement in eldercare]*, Copenhagen: Sundhedsstyrelsen.

Tuntland, H. (2017) *Reablement in Home-Dwelling Older Adults*, Bergen: University of Bergen.

Tuntland, H., Kjeken, I., Folkestad, B., Førland, O., and Langeland, E. (2019) 'Everyday occupations prioritised by older adults participating in reablement: a cross-sectional study', *Scandinavian Journal of Occupational Therapy*, 27(4): 248–58.

van den Bulck, A.O., Metzelthin, S., Elissen, A.M., Stadlander, M.C., Stam, J.E., Wallinga, G., and Ruwaard, D. (2019) 'Which client characteristics predict home-care needs? Results of a survey study among Dutch home-care nurses', *Health & Social Care in the Community*, 27(1): 93–104.

Victorian Department of Human Services (2008) 'Victorian HACC Active Service Model: discussion paper', Melbourne: Victorian Department of Human Services.

Vik, K. (2018) 'Hverdagsrehabilitering og tverrfaglig samarbeid; en empirisk studie i fire norske kommuner', *Tidsskrift for Omsorgsforskning*, 4(1): 6–15.

Wong-Cornall, C., Parsons, J., Sheridan, N., Kenealy, T., and Peckham, A. (2017) 'Extending "continuity of care" to include the contribution of family carers', *International Journal of Integrated Care*, 17(2): 11.

PART II

Outcomes

Does reablement improve client-level outcomes of participants? An investigation of the current evidence

Gill Lewin, John Parsons, Hilary O'Connell, and Silke Metzelthin

Introduction

With ageing populations, reablement is increasingly being seen by governments and service providers as a way of reducing or managing that demand. Some examples of how this has happened in different countries are provided in Chapter 3 by Feiring et al and in Chapter 4 by Parsons et al. The need to reduce or manage the demand for services in order to contain the costs to governments of supporting people as they age and require assistance to remain living in the community, has led many researchers to focus on care costs over time as the primary outcome of interest when examining reablement's effectiveness (Lewin et al, 2013; Lewin et al, 2014; Kjerstad and Tuntland, 2016). In addition to a common belief that ultimately it is the ability to control costs that is important to the government, a great advantage of this research is that the results of different studies are easily comparable. On the other hand, the *client-level outcomes* for program participants, that is, changes that are directly associated with the individual who is engaged in reablement, have often been treated as secondary outcomes only. Further, client-level outcomes have also, as described in Chapter 6 by Tuntland et al, been examined in so many different ways and using so many different patient-reported instruments and standardised tests, that summarising the evidence for reablement's effectiveness at an individual level is very hard. Nevertheless, the primary aim of the present chapter is to do just that – find and summarise the evidence on what individuals gain from participating in reablement as undoubtedly that is what motivates most service providers, their staff, and older people themselves. Its secondary aim is then to consider why the evidence is limited, and how the situation might be improved.

Method

In order to examine the effectiveness of reablement for its participants, it is necessary to first agree on the types of interventions that should be included in an overview of studies, given that as described in, among others, Chapter 2 by Tuntland et al, reablement as an intervention has been called different things in different countries and at different times. It was decided therefore to ignore nomenclature and adopt the methodological approach of the Sims–Gould systematic review by including research that has examined the effectiveness of short-term intensive home-based services which had the express purpose of enabling older people to 'regain or retain the ability to manage some aspects of their care', whether these services were called restorative, reactivation, reablement, or indeed, rehabilitation (2017: 654).

This review includes: (1) all the research and evaluation studies identified by the authors, as well as studies used by the authors of other chapters in this book; (2) which have been published in the last 20 years; and (3) examination of the client-level outcomes for participants. Finally, (4) to ensure that this approach was sufficient in order to identify all relevant studies, the list of identified studies was checked against the reference lists of the seven systematic reviews that have looked at reablement, as well as singular studies subsequently published. Both forward and backward citation searches for the systematic reviews and other key papers were also conducted. No papers published later than 2019 have been included, as this chapter was commenced early in 2020.

Details of the studies examined for our summary can be found in Table 5.1. As is evident in Table 5.1, the studies examined employed a range of methodologies, varying from systematic reviews that included only randomised controlled trials (RCTs), to qualitative studies with no control group, in which the researchers asked participants about their experiences. While there are some differences between evidence hierarchies (University of Canberra, 2021), there is general agreement among health researchers that the strongest evidence of the effectiveness of an intervention (level I) is provided by systematic reviews of methodologically sound (unbiased) RCTs, especially if it has been possible for the researchers to conduct a meta-analysis of the studies' combined data. Single RCTs are then considered to provide only level II, and other controlled studies level III evidence, with the quality of the evidence diminishing with the equivalence of the controls. Case series, cohort, or case–control studies are then considered level IV. While there is less agreement about the hierarchy in the lower levels of evidence, we consider qualitative studies to provide level V evidence. A systematic review that includes level III or IV studies is then considered only able to reflect the level of evidence included. In an attempt to be as inclusive as possible when considering the evidence for reablement having positive outcomes for participants, while the concept of the evidence hierarchy has been used to guide the summary of the current evidence base and the findings of the systematic reviews presented first, the results both of studies published later, as well as early studies not meeting the reviews inclusion criteria, have also been included.

Summary of evidence found

The client-level outcomes that have been most commonly examined are daily functioning, physical function, and quality of life, which is in line with findings in Chapter 6 by Tuntland et al. The evidence relating to each of these outcomes is therefore described in a separate section for each type of outcome, whereas the evidence regarding less commonly examined outcomes is described together in a fourth section.

Daily functioning

One of the most examined individual outcomes is the person's ability to complete the tasks of everyday living. Two types of daily tasks are usually distinguished and measured using different instruments. Activities of Daily Living (ADLs) is a term referring to self-care and mobility such as the ability to shower/bathe, toilet, and get around; while Instrumental Activities of Daily Living (IADLs) refer to tasks related to community-based living such as being able to clean the house, do the laundry, look after finances, make phone calls and so on. How independently people can complete both these types of tasks can be measured objectively by observation or subjectively by self-report. Additionally, a range of measurement instruments has been developed over the years, both for ADLs and IADLs separately and together. It is perhaps therefore not surprising, given the choice available, that a wide range of measures has been used in reablement research as also outlined in the Chapter 6 by Tuntland et al.

Considering first the findings of systematic reviews, which as previously described are considered to provide stronger evidence than a single study, we find the researchers have generally concluded that the evidence for reablement's effectiveness in terms of daily functioning is inconsistent and weak. Whitehead et al (2015) found that only two of the eight studies which measured daily functioning showed a significant improvement in ADL scores in favour of the intervention group compared to the control group – at 3 months (Lewin and Vandermeulen, 2010) and at 12 months (Marek et al, 2006; Lewin and Vandermeulen, 2010). However, two of the studies included in Whitehead et al's review did report that the intervention group improved in a greater number of activities than the control group (Glendinning et al, 2010; Zingmark and Bernspång, 2011). The remaining four studies reviewed

Table 5.1: Studies examined and summary of their results

Systematic reviews

Study reference	Study period	Type of studies included	Studies meeting inclusion criteria	Level of evidence
Cochrane et al, 2016	Not specified	RCTs	2	Level I
Legg et al, 2016	2000 – Feb 2015	RCTs of home care reablement	0	NA
Petterssen and Iwarsson, 2017	2000–14	RCTs, controlled trial, retrospective cohort, pilot non-randomised controlled trial, quasi-experimental, cross-sectional	8	Level III
Sims-Gould et al, 2017	To Aug 2016	RCTs	15	Level I
Tessier et al, 2016	Jan 2001 – Aug 2014	RCTs, controlled trials, data linkage, qualitative	10	Level V
Whitehead et al, 2016	To Nov 2014	RCTs, controlled trials	15	Level III

Studies not included in systematic reviews

Study reference	Study period	Study method	No. subjects	Level of evidence
Beresford et al, 2019b	2016–17	Multicentre Prospective cohort to evaluate different service models	64 with complete data	Level IV
Parsons et al, 2018	2012–14	RCT	183	Level II
Parsons et al, 2019	NA	RCT	403	Level II
Ghatorae, 2013	2012	Client interviews as part of service evaluation	13	Level V
Hjelle et al, 2017	2013–14	Client interviews of participants in Langeland RCT	8	Level V
Langeland et al, 2019	2014–15	Multicentre clinical controlled trial	828	Level III
McGoldrick et al, 2017	2014	Client interviews as part of service evaluation	50	Level V
McLeod and Mair, 2009	2008–9	Client interviews as part of service evaluation	17	Level V

Table 5.1: Studies examined and summary of their results (continued)

Studies not included in systematic reviews

Study reference	Study period	Study method	No. subjects	Level of evidence
Moe, Ingstad and Brataas, 2017	NA	Analysis of staff/client interactions	8	Level V
Parsons et al, 2013	2007–8	Cluster RCT	205	Level II
Reidy et al, 2013	2012	Client interviews as part of service evaluation	13	Level V
Tuntland et al, 2015	2012–14	RCT	61	Level II
Whitehead et al, 2016	2014–15	Feasibility RCT	30	Level II
Wilde and Glendinning, 2012	2010	Client interviews as part of larger mixed-methods study	34	Level V

Note: Levels of evidence: I = systematic reviews of methodologically sound RCTs; II = single methodologically sound RCT; III = controlled trials; IV = case control and cohort studies; V = qualitative studies

(Feldman et al, 1996; Gottlieb and Caro, 2000; Tinetti et al, 2002; Lewin et al, 2013) found only non-significant differences between the intervention and the control group. Similarly, Sims-Gould et al's review (2017) which looked at research conducted up to 8 years later than Whitehead and colleagues, found that only seven of the 15 studies they reviewed, reported beneficial effects in favour of the intervention group. These were: fewer restrictions in daily functioning at 3 months (Melis et al, 2008); improved ADL scores and self-assessed ability in the kitchen at 3 months, and in the execution of domestic tasks at 12 months (Cunliffe et al, 2004); better home management and self-care (Tinetti et al, 2002); improvements in ADL and IADL functioning at 6 months (Courtney et al, 2012) and 12 months (Lewin et al, 2016); better self-perceived performance and satisfaction in the execution of daily tasks at 3 and 9 months (Tuntland et al, 2015), and reduced need for assistance with personal care at 3 and 12 months (Lewin et al, 2013).

Four other and more inclusive systematic reviews were conducted within the period (up to August 2016) covered by Sims-Gould et al (2017). Two of them, Sims-Gould et al (2017) and Whitehead et al (2015), did not restrict themselves to including only RCTs, reviewed many of the same studies as Sims-Gould and therefore had similar findings. Of the seven studies that looked at some aspect of daily function included in the Tessier et al (2016) review, only three showed the intervention group to improve more than the controls. Two of these (Lewin and Vandermeulen, 2010; Parsons et al, 2013) had not been included in the Sims-Gould review. Similarly, Pettersson and Iwarsson (2017) found only three of the eight studies they reviewed measured any aspect of daily function, but two of them showed greater improvement in ADLs in the intervention group than the control group. One of these, the study by Winkel et al (2015), had also not been included in the Sims-Gould review and showed the significant ADL gains made by the intervention group were sustained over 12 months. The other two reviews that examined the research happening within a similar period, both adopted the inclusion criterion of the study needing to be an RCT. Legg et al (2016) was more restrictive in the approach, and wished to look only at studies of home care reablement, and as a result, were unable to identify any studies that met their criteria. They therefore concluded that there was no evidence for the effectiveness of home care reablement. This has sometimes been mistakenly interpreted as 'evidence that it is not effective' rather than simply that currently there is a lack of evidence. Cochrane et al (2016), on the other hand, found two RCTs that met their inclusion criteria, Lewin et al (2013) and Tuntland et al (2015) (both also included in the Sims-Gould review) and conducted a meta-analysis of their combined data. The reviewers concluded that there is evidence that reablement slightly improves daily functioning in the short-term (3 months) (both studies) and long-term (9 months) (Tuntland et al, 2015) and 12 months (Lewin et al, 2013) as compared to usual care, but that the evidence is of poor quality as both studies (especially the Lewin one) had the potential for bias because of issues with the methodology.

Research on reablement has, if anything, gained pace and rigour since the systematic reviews discussed previously were completed, and there have been a number of RCTs (Whitehead et al, 2016; Parsons et al, 2017; Parsons et al, 2018; Parsons et al, 2019), clinical controlled trials (Langeland et al, 2019) and cohort studies (McGoldrick et al, 2017; Slater and Hasson, 2018; Beresford et al, 2019a, 2019b) looking at daily functioning. The results for effectiveness in ADL or daily functioning have again been mixed.

Parsons et al's (2017) RCT showed no significant differences in daily functioning between the intervention and control group over 24 months of follow-up. In another RCT conducted by Parsons et al (2018) participants in the intervention group were significantly less dependent in bathing and dressing the lower body after 6 months than participants in the control group. However, there were no differences between the groups in relation to any other of the ADL and IADL activities. A third RCT conducted by Parsons and colleagues in 2019 found no significant differences between the intervention and control group after 12 months. In the non-randomised controlled trial of Langeland et al (2019) there were significant treatment effects in favour of the intervention group at 10 weeks and 6 months follow-up. However, the effect had disappeared by 12 months.

In a cohort study by Beresford and colleagues (2019a, 2019b), there was a statistically significant improvement in ADL score between baseline and first follow-up at 6 months, and in both ADL and IADL scores between baseline and the second follow-up 6 months later. The difference in scores between first and second follow-ups was significant for IADL functioning only. In the retrospective cohort study of Slater and Hasson (2018), a statistically significant improvement in daily functioning was found after 15 months. In the small-scale feasibility study of Whitehead et al (2016), the intervention group seemed to improve more regarding daily functioning compared to the control group, although for personal ADLs this was most obvious at 2 weeks whereas the difference on IADLs was not evident until 3 months. Finally, a cohort study conducted to evaluate the Befriending and Reablement Service (BARS) in the UK (McGoldrick et al, 2017) reported that their results clearly indicated the benefits of reablement in sustaining and improving older people's capacity for independent living. However, due to it being an uncontrolled pre-post service evaluation with self-report measures, the findings cannot be considered to provide reliable evidence.

Summing up, the evidence for the effectiveness of reablement with regard to functioning in ADL is weak and where an intervention effect is found in the shorter term, it is not always sustained in the longer term (Beresford et al, 2019a, 2019b; Langeland et al, 2019). An additional view relating to the impact of reablement on daily functioning is provided by a systematic review by Buma et al (2022) and which is not considered in depth in this chapter due to the recency of its publication. Buma et al's (2022) systematic review of 20 RCTs and CCTs included two studies not considered in the systematic reviews presented in this chapter (Szanton et al, 2019; Roojackers et al, 2021).

Physical function

Physical function underpins an individual's ability to perform many everyday activities of daily living. For example, being independent in showering requires mobility, strength, balance, and some flexibility. Physical function measures are, however, often independent of the everyday activity for which they are required. They also most commonly involve practitioners' observation of performance in physical tasks rather than users' self-report, although not in all cases. Two common measures are the Timed Up and Go (TUG), a test of mobility, which measures the time it takes an individual to get up from a chair and cover a specified distance with or without an aid (Podsiadlo and Richardson, 1991), and the Short Physical Performance Battery (SPPB) which comprises a test of standing balance, a timed 4 metre walk test, and a timed test of five repetitions of rising from a chair and sitting down (Guralnik et al, 1994).

As mentioned in the introduction to this chapter, client-level outcomes, in general, have often been considered secondary to outcomes such as service use. Furthermore, different aspects of physical function have often only been included as supplementary to other client-level outcomes such as functional dependence and quality of life, rather than being the main focus of effectiveness studies. This is also true for the four systematic reviews that considered any measures of physical ability or activity at all, as none considered physical function as the primary outcome of interest (Whitehead et al, 2015; Tessier et al, 2016; Pettersson and Iwarsson, 2017; Sims-Gould et al, 2017).

The Tessier et al (2016), Pettersson and Iwarsson (2017), and Sims-Gould et al (2017) reviews all found that mobility was the physical function outcome examined most often, although measured in a variety of ways. The TUG, already described, was the most common measure and was used in four separate studies, only one of which showed a significant intervention effect according to Sims-Gould et al (2017). However, the study referred to, although finding a very significant improvement in TUG scores especially at the 1-year follow up for the small sample that received the intervention, did not have a contemporary control group. Instead, it compared the outcomes with those from an earlier trial of the service delivery model in which health professionals had delivered the intervention, rather than non-health professionals (Lewin et al, 2016). Of the other three studies, two found that both intervention and control groups' TUG scores improved, whereas the third found no change (Melis et al, 2008; Comans et al, 2010; Tuntland et al, 2015).

The other measures of mobility in studies included in one or more of the systematic reviews have relied on users' self-report, which although potentially less reliable, could be considered to be more meaningful in terms of how an individual sees their own life being affected by the intervention. Courtney et al (2012) used a walking impairment scale and found that in comparison to the control group, the intervention group reported greater improvements over time in their ability to walk longer distances, the speed they were able to walk, and in the number of stairs they could climb without difficulty, while Tinetti and colleagues (2002) asked about an individual's self-reported ability to walk and transfer from bed to chair, and found that individuals who had received restorative home care reported a small but significantly greater improvement than recipients of standard home care.

Another measure of physical function that has been used in a number of different studies is the physical function scale of the Short Form 36 (SF36) Health Survey. Whitehead et al (2015) as part of their systematic review, looked at the results of this scale for the five studies that had met their inclusion criteria, and had used the SF36. They found that two of the studies showed the improvement in the intervention group to be significantly different from the control (Markle-Reid, 2002; Parsons et al, 2012), and while none of the other three studies found a statistical difference between intervention and control, the results favoured the intervention group in all three (Markle-Reid et al, 2006: Markle-Reid et al, 2011; King et al, 2012).

A further study included in two of the systematic reviews, Burton et al (2013), used a self-report measure to look at the overall physical activity levels of home care recipients, some of whom had participated in the Home Independence Program (HIP), a restorative/reablement) program, also described in Chapter 3 by Feiring et al and in Chapter 4 by Parsons et al, while others had just received traditional home care. The HIP group was found to be significantly more active, as reported on the Physical Activity Scale for the Elderly (PASE). However, when other variables were included in a logistic regression, participation in the HIP group was not found to be a predictor of activity level. This result prompted a trial comparing the traditional exercise program originally used within HIP to a Lifestyle Exercise program (LiFe) based around common everyday activities (Burton et al, 2014). Participants completing LiFe showed significant improvements on 25 per cent of the physical function measures at follow up, whereas no significant gains were shown on any measures by participants in the original structured exercise program.

An exception to the generalisation that physical function is only looked at as an adjunct to other outcomes was the cluster randomised controlled trial conducted by Parsons and colleagues in New Zealand (2013) included in the Sims-Gould and Tessier reviews where physical function measured by the Short Physical Performance Battery (SPPB) was one of the main outcome measures. That study found at 6 months follow up that the restorative home care group showed a significantly greater improvement in their overall SPPB score and in the gait speed component of the scale, as compared to the control group, who received traditional home care. However, the differences between the intervention and control groups' baseline and follow up scores on the balance and chair-stand components were not significant. Despite the apparently positive result in terms of the total SPPB score, the authors expressed some concern that the degree of improvement shown by the intervention group was not large enough to be clinically meaningful, and that more emphasis is needed on assisting restorative home care participants to mobilise safely in the community, as the lack of this ability was thought to have been a factor in the study, also finding that there was not the hoped for improvement in social support.

A study that due to its relative recency was not included in any of the systematic reviews and used the SSPB to look at physical activity as a secondary outcome, was a clinical controlled trial (CCT) conducted in Norway by Langeland et al (2019). Despite their findings being more positive than the New Zealand study, they were still mixed. Authors found a significantly positive effect of reablement on all measures at 10 weeks and 6 months compared to a control group, but the effect for balance and walking was lost at 12 months, although still evident for the overall score and the sit-to-stand measure. Especially notable was the fact that the improvement shown in the total score was greater than 1 and therefore of sufficient size to meet the most stringent criterion for clinical significance discussed by Parsons et al (2013).

In summary, studies included in the systematic reviews that used measures of physical function have shown mixed results. None of the reviewers had identified the assessment of reablement's effectiveness in terms of physical function as a primary outcome, only the Sims–Gould et al (2017) review made specific reference to it in their discussion where they reported that there was evidence that mobility could be improved, and deterioration delayed. The subsequently conducted CCT by Langeland et al (2019) can be seen as providing partial support for these contentions in relation to mobility, as balance and walking improved significantly in the first 6 months but not in the next 6, while sit-to-stand and the overall SPPB score showed an intervention effect at 12 months.

Quality of life

As described in relation to the previous outcomes, QoL has usually not been the prime outcome of interest. Additionally, as with daily activities and physical function, there is considerable variation in how QoL has been measured, both in the studies included in the systematic reviews and in other articles not included in the reviews. However, whereas for daily functioning and physical function there is a commonality between the tools in how they understand what is being looked at, that is not necessarily true for QoL, as different tools can include quite different domains. For example, the SF-36 and EQ-5D-5L, the two most used tools in the studies examined for this chapter, describe themselves as measuring health-related quality of life (HRQoL). The SF-36 explores eight health concepts: vitality; physical functioning; bodily pain; general health perceptions; physical role functioning; emotional role functioning; social role functioning, and mental health (Ware and Sherbourne, 1992), while the EQ-5D-5L includes only five domains – mobility, self-care, usual activities, pain/discomfort, and anxiety/depression (Herdman et al, 2011). Other tools that have been used do not define themselves as health-related and include Assessment of Quality of Life (AQOL) scale used in the study by Lewin et al (2013), COOP/Wonka in the study by Tuntland et al (2015), and the Adult Social Care Outcomes Toolkit (ASCOT) in the study by Beresford et al (2019). However, despite the different construction and conceptualisation of quality of life within the tools making it difficult to interpret the outcome for the individuals involved, there is still developing evidence that demonstrates the impact of reablement on this important service user outcome.

Five of the eight studies included in the Whitehead et al (2015) systematic review that looked at QoL used the SF–36, and all five found a significant improvement in HRQoL for the reablement group as compared to the controls. The two New Zealand based RCTs (King et al, 2012; Parsons et al, 2012), as well as the two RCTs from Canada (Markle-Reid et al, 2002; Markle-Reid et al, 2006), demonstrated significant changes in SF–36 scores at the 6-month follow-up, while the UK study of 1,015 adults aged 18 and over who received reablement services found that the improvement was sustained over a 9- to 12-month follow-up (Glendinning et al, 2010). Of the other three studies in the review, one found no difference between the intervention and control, while follow-up data was not available in the other two.

The Sims-Gould et al (2017) systematic review identified two studies that had looked at quality of life. Whereas one of them, the Dutch EASYCare study, found a significant difference between the intervention group and control over the 6 months of follow-up on the Medical Health Outcomes Study – mental health subscale (Melis et al, 2008), the other, an RCT conducted in Norway by Tuntland and colleagues (2015), found no significant difference between the groups on the COOP/Wonka, a generic self-report scale.

Four of the studies included in Tessier et al's (2016) review looked at QoL. While all four found the improvement in the intervention group to be larger than in the control group, the difference was only significant in three studies. All four of these studies had also been included in Whitehead et al's (2015) review and the three that found the significant intervention effect had used the SF-36 (Glendinning et al, 2010; King et al, 2012; Parsons et al, 2012) whereas Lewin et al (2013) had used the Assessment of Quality of Life (AQOL) scale and found no difference between the group that received the reablement intervention and the group that received standard home care. Three of these four studies were also included in the Pettersson and Iwarsson (2017) systematic review (King et al, 2012; Parsons et al, 2012; Lewin et al, 2013). Additionally, their review included the study by Burton and her colleagues (2013) which found a significant difference in the physical component score of the SF-12 between individuals who had received a reablement service and those who had received a standard home care service.

Finally, the Cochrane systematic review which had stricter inclusion criteria than any of the others included only the Lewin et al (2013) and Tuntland et al (2015) studies; neither of which found a significant intervention effect on their QOL measures. However, it is worth noting that all studies that used the SF-36 or SF-12 to measure HRQoL found a significant change over time when reablement was compared to a control/usual care group. Additionally, this improvement was observed by carers of the older people randomised to receive reablement in the New Zealand based RCT by Senior et al (2014).

In contrast to this consistency in results using different versions of the SF Survey, a range of results have been evident when different versions of the EuroQoL have been used. A New Zealand based RCT with 113 participants found no difference between the intervention and control groups using the EuroQoL thermometer visual analogue scale (Parsons et al, 2017), while a clinical controlled trial of 707 older people in Norway with assessments using EQ-5D-5L at baseline, after 10 weeks and then at 6 and 12 months found significant improvements at 3 and 6 months on only some of the subscales (mobility, personal care, usual activities, and current health status) and they were not sustained at the 1-year follow up (Langeland et al, 2019). A lack of sustained improvement was also found by Beresford et al (2019), in an observational cohort study of 143 UK based reablement services. While a significant change in EQ-5D-5L between admission and discharge from the service was shown, it was not sustained by the time of the 6-month follow-up. An identical finding was also observed in the pattern of ASCOT data with an initial improvement in index scores that was not sustained at the 6-month follow-up.

In summary, there is inconclusive evidence of the impact of reablement on QoL among older people. It is suggested that this may be partly due to the different tools used to measure this complex phenomenon. Although promising results are reported in robust studies that have used the SF-36, these are not supported by studies that have used other tools to measure QoL. In addition, where longer follow-up periods have been used, it would appear that improvements may not be sustained.

Other client-level outcomes

Although not many other client-level outcomes have been included in effectiveness studies, there is, as with the more common outcomes already discussed, variation in the types of measures used. Whereas research studies have used different standardised outcome tools, service evaluations, which are uncontrolled and therefore provide a lower level of evidence, generally have used either tools they have developed themselves or have used recognised outcome measures in a non-standard manner.

Just two systematic reviews examined the findings related to client-level outcomes other than the three outcomes already discussed. The Whitehead et al (2015) review included five studies that looked at depression/mood as a secondary outcome. Only two studies found a significant intervention effect, and both of these used the Centers for Epidemiological Studies Depression Scale (CESD) (Markle-Reid, 2002; Markle-Reid et al, 2006). However, the two others that used the CESD found no effect, nor did the study that used Mood indicators – Minimum dataset (Whitehead et al, 2015, Appendix 2). Another psychosocial measure identified in the Whitehead review was morale, measured using the Philadelphia Geriatric Centre Morale Scale (PGCMS). A significant intervention effect was found by the study reviewed by Whitehead (Lewin and Vandermeulen, 2010), but not by either of the two studies cited in the Sims–Gould et al (2017) review as having used this measure (Martin et al, 1994; Donald et al, 1995).

Other outcomes measured in studies included in the Sims–Gould et al (2017) review were cognition, pain, and social support. No significant intervention effects were found for any of these outcomes. Nor was any impact found on social support as measured by the Duke Social Support Index in a separate New Zealand study of the restorative home support model (Parsons et al, 2013). Another outcome noted by Sims–Gould et al (2017) was the increase in falls found for the intervention group by Comans and colleagues (2010). In contrast, a small feasibility randomised controlled trial conducted by Whitehead and colleagues (2016) found a significant reduction in falls in the intervention group compared to the controls.

As already noted, service evaluations have often not used standardised client-level outcome measures, but where they have, they have used measures especially relevant for the particular client group targeted by the service. Thus, in their evaluation of the Southwark Reablement service, Reidy and colleagues (2013) used the Warwick Edinburgh Mental Health Wellbeing Scale (WEMWBS) because the service is targeted at people with mental health issues. However, only nine of the 67 service recipients participating in the evaluation completed pre- and post- data collection, and although there was a small mean improvement in their scores, the numbers were too small for this to be statistically significant. Other measures used by Reidy et al (2013) included the Health of the Nation Outcome Scale (HONOS) and assessment on the Fair Access to Care Services (FACS) Criteria, which was used as the basis for eligibility for the service. Individuals had to be assessed as having substantial or moderate needs to be accepted by the service. No significant improvement was shown on the HONOS following the 13-week service period, but there was a significant overall decrease in the FACS criteria with 33 people moving from the substantial to moderate needs category. There was a significant change during reablement in six of the 12 FACS dimensions. These were: community and isolation; safety indoors; decision making; personal care – hygiene; work and learning; home – domestic routines.

Other studies that have used standardised measures have been multi-site studies conducted by researchers, rather than service evaluations commissioned by the service itself. In England, Beresford and colleagues (2019) looked at three statutorily funded reablement services using a battery of outcome measures including functional dependency and quality of life measures already discussed. In addition, they used the General Health Questionnaire (GHQ-12) to see whether reablement participants reported changes in their mental health following reablement. The mean scores at the 12 weeks and 6 months follow-ups were significantly improved compared to the mean baseline scores with just over two-thirds of individuals (68 per cent) having an improved score at 6 months, while equal proportions (16 per cent) had deteriorated or had the same score as baseline.

Another multi-site study conducted by researchers, but this time in Norway (Langeland et al, 2019), looked at individuals' sense of coherence as a secondary outcome, on the basis that reablement is a health-promoting approach, and sense of coherence is a central concept in certain theories of health promotion. Using the Sense of Coherence questionnaire (SOC-13), a self-report measure which has been judged as 'a reliable, valid and cross-culturally applicable instrument for measuring how people manage stress and stay well' (Eriksson and Lindstrom, 2005: 460), the researchers found a significant intervention effect at 6 months, which was then no longer significant at the 12-month follow-up (Langeland et al, 2019).

Two evaluations frequently referred to in the literature, examined reablement services in cities in Scotland. The first, conducted by McLeod and Mair (2009), had an experimental design and included a control group, whereas the second, by Ghatorae (2013), was a small observational cohort study. Both included follow-up interviews of participants to ask about their reablement experience. Ghatorae's study (2013) also included a survey to enable quantification of the numbers achieving specified outcomes. McLeod and Mair (2009) found a high rate of satisfaction with participants' reduced need for services with many saying that it helped them get back on their feet and they could not have coped without the service. Ghatorae's study also found a high rate of satisfaction with 84 per cent saying they could resume usual activities, 74 per cent that they could do more for themselves and 56 per cent that they needed less support following the program (2013).

A later United Kingdom service evaluation (McGoldrick et al, 2017), used what they called the STAR tool for self-assessment plus an interview based on the Adult Social Care Outcomes Toolkit (ASCOT), to look at outcomes. The ASCOT is a multi-faceted preference weighted measure of social care quality of life outcomes developed in the UK (Netten et al, 2002). In response to the ASCOT interview, the results indicated there had been improvements in safety, meals and nutrition, activities/occupation, control over daily life, social participating, accommodation cleanliness and comfort, dignity and respect, as well as in anxiety levels. The study however was an observational cohort with no control group and small samples, and no data was included in the report, only bar charts (McGoldrick et al, 2014; McGoldrick et al, 2017).

While generally, studies that have included a measure of participant satisfaction have found participants to be satisfied with reablement, this was not the case in the Feldman et al study (1996), reviewed by Whitehead et al (2015), as these researchers found user satisfaction to be significantly lower in the intervention group than the control.

In addition to studies designed to evaluate the effectiveness of specific reablement services, a number of researchers have conducted separate qualitative studies to throw light on users' experience and perceptions of reablement services. Thus, Wilde and Glendinning (2012) conducted a study using a case series approach and found that while most participants felt they had benefitted from reablement and made gains in their ADLs and IADLs, their social needs were being insufficiently considered.

Two more recent qualitative case series studies both conducted in Norway have provided important insights into the factors that influence variation in individuals' 'success' with reablement, Hjelle et al (2017) and Moe et al (2017). Such studies are important as even in those trials where a significantly better outcome for reablement participants compared to controls has been shown, there is variation between individuals, and it is very unusual for all participants to have equally good outcomes. Similarly, even in those trials which find no significant differences between people who have participated in reablement and people who have not, there are individuals who have made significant gains whose achievements are not acknowledged as they are hidden within the average insignificant result.

Summarising, there is again little consistent and robust evidence for the effectiveness of reablement in terms of client-level outcomes as measured by the various formal tools used. This is despite apparently high levels of satisfaction and self-reported positive outcomes in service-level evaluations. Whether this apparent discrepancy reflects the inappropriateness of the outcomes being measured or that interventions delivered as part of a rigorously controlled research trial cannot be as individually tailored as needed to optimise outcomes, will be discussed in the next section.

Discussion

The aim of this chapter was to summarise the evidence on what individuals gain from participating in reablement. The evidence that individuals show greater improvement in client-level outcomes following reablement rather than traditional home care is still very limited and it can be argued that the situation has changed little since the review by Ryburn and her colleagues (2009). At that time, they pointed to an emerging body of evidence that restorative approaches in home care, including reablement, may result in greater improvement in function and quality of life than traditional home care. Subsequent research findings have been mixed, and the quality of evidence generally poor, apart perhaps from the evidence regarding QoL. Only one of the systematic reviews had a very positive conclusion regarding client-level outcomes and this was about HRQoL: "There is good evidence supporting the effectiveness of reablement particularly regarding HRQoL and service utilisation" (Tessier et al, 2016: 56).

Other reviewers were less positive about reablement's effectiveness: "4R interventions show some promise in the home care context" (Sims-Gould et al, 2017: 661).

> there is *some scientific support* indicating that this type of intervention or program has a potential to provide positive effects ... there are several indications of positive effects on primary outcomes such as reduced need home/hospital care, remaining living at home and health related quality of life. Also, secondary outcomes such as improved independence in ADL, increased physical activity, and improved physical health, as well as reduced costs, seem promising. (Pettersson and Iwarsson, 2017: 282)

> Overall, there is *some evidence* that interventions aiming to improve ability to independently perform ADL are effective for a population of home-care service users. ... There is *also some evidence* that these interventions improve health related quality of life. (Whitehead et al, 2015: 1073)

> The findings of this review were based on two studies and the evidence was uniformly very low quality for all outcomes. From the results of meta-analyses of the two included studies, reablement may slightly improve functional status but may have little or no effect on QoL. (Cochrane et al, 2016: 20)

The available evidence for the effect of reablement on the daily functioning of service recipients is weak, with any positive impact only being sustainable over a short term. For physical functioning, there is inconclusive evidence of the effect of reablement, with some evidence that mobility could be improved, and deterioration delayed. The lack of a consistent tool to measure QoL has resulted in some evidence for a positive change in SF-36 scores in several studies, but this is not shown in studies that have used other tools to measure this important construct. Finally, there is an absence of robust evidence for the effect of reablement on other client-level outcomes.

While the results from service evaluations are in the main more positive, especially as regards satisfaction with the service, the evidence most provide can only be considered weak due to one or more of the following characteristics: a lack of a control/comparison group, the use of unstandardised data collection and tools, and the evaluators being aware of what services someone had received when they collected outcome data.

There are several issues underlying our current lack of what would be considered a robust evidence base. The first issue was a *lack of an agreed definition of reablement*. Although this has recently been addressed through the publication of an international definition achieved through consensus by reablement researchers and experts (Metzelthin et al, 2020), this means that it has not always been clear that we are all talking about the same thing when we discuss the effectiveness of reablement, and try to compare or synthesise the results of different studies (as also described in Chapter 6 by Tuntland et al). For instance, Legg et al (2016), concluded that there was no evidence for the effectiveness of home care reablement, on the basis that no studies met their inclusion criteria for their systematic review. The criterion that studies could not meet was being a randomised controlled trial of reablement provided by home care workers not operating within the context of a multidisciplinary team, a service delivery model common in the UK but rare in other parts of the world. Although undoubtedly an issue when trying to build an evidence-base, the differences between reablement service models can be seen as reflecting the different histories and political and service contexts of their development in different countries, as illustrated in Chapter 3 by Feiring et al and in Chapter 4 by Parsons et al. The resulting differences in service models can then be seen as quite legitimate and appropriate, at least until there is overwhelming evidence that a particular service model/models result in substantially better outcomes for individuals and could be adapted to most contexts, perhaps also because reablement itself embraces the concept of the need to tailor interventions to a particular individual and their circumstances, and thus complies with current perspectives of person-centredness and empowerment.

Ascertainment of the comparative effectiveness of different models brings us to the second issue – the *diversity of outcome measures and types of outcomes* that have so far been used. As described in detail in Chapter 6 by Tuntland et al, and illustrated in the present chapter, not only are many different tools used to measure the individual outcomes most examined, but there is no apparent agreement on the types of individual outcomes that reablement is designed to help the individual achieve. The lack of an agreed set of standardised outcome measures makes a systematic review of the evidence very hard, and meta-analyses impossible or extremely limited, and thus limits our ability to answer the question addressed by this chapter.

Both of the aforementioned difficulties could perhaps be addressed by *greater collaboration and discussion between stakeholders* (such as policy makers, service providers, and researchers) across the world in order to agree on the critical elements of a reablement service model and a set of outcome measures to measure its effectiveness. This has essentially been achieved in relation to falls prevention by the work of PROFANE (Prevention of Falls Network Europe), who have not only developed a consensus statement on defining and measuring falls, but also developed a taxonomy of falls prevention interventions. The activities of the ReAble Network, many of whom are authors included in this book, are centred around achieving such consensus, as described on the network website, https://reable.auckl and.ac.nz/.

When considering the process for achieving such consensus it is *essential to involve all stakeholders*. Users of reablement services need to be involved in the determination of the domains (and accompanying tools/measures) that are most appropriate to use to measure the impact of reablement services at a personal level. Policy makers and service providers need also to be involved, as researchers cannot conduct rigorous trials without sufficient funding to implement a new service or without there being existing services that can be defined as reablement. When it is considered that reablement is a relatively new approach, it is hardly surprising that there have been few RCTs and even fewer in which all aspects of the methodology have been sufficiently well controlled to be considered free of bias and to therefore provide strong evidence. Reablement needs to be embedded into a service system for this type of research to be conducted, and such implementation is complex, time-consuming and costly as it requires not only training/ retraining staff but changing the culture of the service organisations and staff and the expectations of service recipients and their families. As yet, few countries have attempted this. The effectiveness of a complex intervention such as reablement, is critically influenced by its implementation within the local and national context, and without agreed mechanisms for describing service models, their implementation and daily operation, as well as how effectiveness is measured, it will not be possible to provide a definitive answer to the question of whether reablement works on an individual level for its participants.

The importance of context when looking at reablement implementation was emphasised by the results of a very recent study by Jacobi et al (2020) which examined the relationship between personal and neighbourhood characteristics and reablement success defined as reduced service use. While individual differences in reablement outcomes have been recognised in many service evaluations, only a small number of previous studies (Newbronner et al, 2007; Wilde and Glendinning, 2012; Lewin et al, 2013) had attempted to identify those characteristics that predicted success, and their findings were not entirely consistent. Looking at the data from ten thousand plus individuals who had received reablement in Essex County in the UK over a 4-year period, they found that not only are some personal characteristics such as level of disability, age and prior service use associated with a reduced likelihood of reablement success, but their effect is potentiated by neighbourhood variables measuring deprivation and level of crime. This study's authors concluded that reablement services could potentially be more successful if tailored to client groups and to specific geo-demographic contexts.

Conclusion

The evidence that reablement enables older adults to have better client-level outcomes than if they had only received traditional home care, can still only be considered weak, although in relation to outcomes such as quality of life or wellbeing, perhaps promising. On the other hand, it was extremely rare for outcomes to have been found to be worse for reablement participants, no difference being the common finding, and user satisfaction has generally been found to be high. If, therefore, the findings regarding reablement's effectiveness in reducing services use are robust, should the question then be whether a lack of robust evidence for better client-level outcomes should influence the adoption of reablement into a service system? In these times of population ageing an approach that reduces the demand for aged care services and does not negatively impact on individuals' health, function, and wellbeing, is surely a better use of public money than one which will need ever-increasing funding, as demand is fuelled by increasing numbers of elders. More research is, however, needed on how services or service systems can be tailored for specific groups and contexts, in order to maximise reablement's effectiveness.

References

Beresford, B., Mayhew, E., Duarte, A., Faria, R., Weatherly, H., Mann, R., Parker, G., Aspinal, F., and Kanaan, M. (2019a) 'Outcomes of reablement and their measurement: findings from an evaluation of English reablement services', *Health & Social Care in the Community*, 27: 1438–50.

Beresford, B., Mann, R., Parker, G., Kanaan, M., Fariam R., Rabiee, P., Weatherly, H., Clarke, S., Mayhew, E., Duarte, A., Laver-Fawcett A., and Aspinal, F. (2019b) 'Reablement services for people at risk of needing social care: the MoRe mixed-methods evaluation', *Health Services Delivery Research*, 7(16).

Buma, L.E., Vluggen, S., Zwakhalen, S., Kempen, G.I., and Metzelthin, S. (2022) 'Effects on clients' daily functioning and common features of reablement interventions: a systematic literature review', *European Journal of Ageing*, 1–27.

Burton, E., Lewin, G., and Boldy, D. (2013) 'Physical activity levels of older people receiving a home care service', *Journal of Aging and Physical Activity*, 21(2): 140–54.

Burton, E., Lewin, G., Clemson, L., and Boldy, D. (2014) 'Long term benefits of a lifestyle exercise program for older people receiving a restorative home care service: a pragmatic randomized controlled trial', *Healthy Aging & Clinical Care in the Elderly*, 6: 1–9.

Cochrane, A., Furlong, M., McGilloway, S., Molloy, D.W., Stevenson, M., and Donnelly, M. (2016) 'Time-limited home-care reablement services for maintaining and improving the functional independence of older adults', *Cochrane Database of Systematic Reviews*, Issue 10, Art. No.: CD010825.

Comans, T.A., Brauer, S.G., and Haines, T.P. (2010) 'Randomized trial of domiciliary versus center-based rehabilitation: which is more effective in reducing falls and improving quality of life in older fallers?', *Journal of Gerontology Series A: Biological Sciences and Medical Sciences*, 65: 672–9.

Courtney, M.D., Edwards, H.E., Chang, A.M., Parker, A.W., Finlayson, K., Bradbury, C., and Nielsen, Z. (2012) 'Improved functional ability and independence in activities of daily living for older adults at high risk of hospital readmission: a randomized controlled trial', *Journal of Evaluation in Clinical Practice*, 18: 128–34.

Cunliffe, A.L., Gladman, J.R., Husbands, S.L., Miller, P., Dewey, M.E., and Harwood, R.H. (2004) 'Sooner and healthier: a randomised controlled trial and interview study of an early discharge rehabilitation service for older people', *Age and Ageing*, 33(3): 246–52.

Donald, I.P., Baldwin, R.N., and Bannerjee, M. (1995) 'Gloucester hospital-at-home: a randomized controlled trial', *Age and Ageing*, 24: 434–9.

Eriksson, M. and Lindström, B. (2005) 'Validity of Antonovsky's sense of coherence scale: a systematic review', *Journal of Epidemiology and Community Health*, 59(6): 460–6.

Feldman, P.H., Latimer, E., and Davidson, H. (1996) 'Medicaid funded home care for the frail elderly and disabled: evaluating the cost savings and outcomes of a service delivery reform', *Health Services Research*, 31(4): 489–513.

Ghatorae, H. (2013) *Reablement in Glasgow: Quantitative and Qualitative Research*, Glasgow: Glasgow City Council.

Glendinning, C., Jones, K., Baxter, K., Rabiee, P., Curtis, L.A., Wilde, A., Arksey, H., and Forder, J.E. (2010) *Home Care Re-ablement Services: Investigating the Longer Term Impacts (Prospective Longitudinal Study)*, York: Social Policy Research Unit, University of York.

Gottlieb, A. and Caro, F. (2000) 'Providing low-tech assistive equipment through home care services: the Massachusetts Assistive Equipment Demonstration', *Technology and Disability*, 13: 41–53.

Guralnik, J.M., Simonsick, E.M., Ferrucci, L., Glynn, R.J., Berkman, L.F., Blazer, D.G., Sherr, P.A., and Wallace, R.B. (1994) 'A short physical performance battery assessing lower extremity function: association with self-reported disability and prediction of mortality and nursing home admission', *Journal of Gerontology*, 49(2): M85–94.

Herdman, M., Gudex, C., Lloyd, A., Janssen, M., Kind, P., Parkin, D., Bonsel, G. and Badia, X. (2011) 'Development and preliminary testing of the new five-level version of EQ-5D (EQ-5D-5L)', *Quality of Life Research*, 20(10): 1727–36.

Hjelle, K.M., Tuntland, H., Førland, O., and Alvsvåg, H. (2017) 'Driving forces for home-based reablement; a qualitative study of older adults' experiences', *Health & Social Care in the Community*, 25(5): 1581–9.

Jacobi, C.J., Thiel, D., and Allum, N. (2020) 'Enabling and constraining successful reablement: individual and neighbourhood factors', *PLoS ONE*, 15(9): e0237432.

King, A., Parsons, M., and Robinson, E. (2012) 'Assessing the impact of a restorative home care service in New Zealand: a cluster randomised controlled trial', *Health & Social Care in the Community*, 20: 365–74.

Kjerstad, E. and Tuntland, H.K. (2016) 'Reablement in community-dwelling older adults: a cost-effectiveness analysis alongside a randomized controlled trial', *Health Economics Review*, 12(6): 1–10.

Langeland, E., Tuntland, H., Folkestad, B., Førland, O., Jacobsen, F.F., and Kjeken, I. (2019) 'A multicenter investigation of reablement in Norway: a clinical controlled trial', *BMC Geriatrics*, 19(29).

Legg, L., Gladman, J., Drummond, A., and Davidson, A. (2016) 'A systematic review of the evidence on home care reablement services', *Clinical Rehabilitation*, 30(8): 741–9.

Lewin, G. and Vandermeulen, S. (2010) 'A non-randomised controlled trial of the Home Independence Program (HIP): an Australian restorative programme for older home-care clients', *Health & Social Care in the Community*, 18: 91–9.

Lewin, G., De San Miguel, K., Knuiman, M., Alan, J., Boldy, D., Hendrie, D., and Vandermeulen, S. (2013) 'A randomised controlled trial of the Home Independence Program, an Australian restorative home-care programme for older adults', *Health & Social Care in the Community*, 21: 69–78.

Lewin, G., Allan, J., Patterson, C., Knuiman, M., Boldy, D., and Hendrie, D. (2014) 'A comparison of the home-care and healthcare service use and costs of older Australians randomised to receive a restorative or a conventional home-care service', *Health & Social Care in the Community*, 22(3): 328–36.

Lewin, G., Concanen, K., and Youens, D. (2016) 'The Home Independence Program with non-health professionals as care managers: an evaluation', *Clinical Interventions in Aging*, 11: 807–17.

Marek, K.D., Popejoy, L., Petroski, G., and Rantz, M. (2006) 'Nurse care coordination in community-based long-term care', *Journal of Nursing Scholarship*, 38: 80–6.

Markle-Reid, M. (2002) *Frail Elderly Home Care Clients: The Effects and Expense of Adding Nursing Health Promotion and Preventive Care to Personal Support Services*, Ontario Canada: Macmaster University.

Markle-Reid, M., Weir, R., Browne, G., Roberts, J., Gafni, A., and Henderson, S. (2006) 'Health promotion for frail older home care clients', *Journal of Advanced Nursing*, 54: 381–95.

Markle-Reid, M., Orridge, C.R., Weir, G.B., Browne, G., Gafni, A., Lewis, M., Walsh, M., Levy, C., Daub, S., Brien, H., Roberts, J., and Thabane, L. (2011) 'Interprofessional stroke rehabilitation for stroke survivors using home care', *Canadian Journal of Neurological Sciences*, 38(2): 317–34.

Martin, F., Oyewole, A., and Moloney, A. (1994) 'A randomized controlled trial of a high support hospital discharge team for elderly people', *Age and Ageing*, 23: 228–34.

McGoldrick, C., McEvoy, D., and Barrett, G. (2014) *Evaluation of BARS: Befriending and Re-ablement Service in Sefton*, Liverpool: The Centre for the Study of Crime, Criminalisation and Social Exclusion, Liverpool John Moores University.

McGoldrick, C., Barrett, G.A., and Cook, I. (2017) 'Befriending and re-ablement service: a better alternative in an age of austerity', *International Journal of Sociology and Social Policy*, 37(1/2): 51–68.

McLeod, B., Mair, M., and RP&M Associates (2009) *Evaluation of City of Edinburgh Council Home Care Re-Ablement Service*, Edinburgh: Scottish Government Social Research.

Melis, R.J., Van Eijken, M.I., Teerenstra, S., Van Achterberg, T., Parker, S.G., Borm, G.F., Van de Lisdonk, E.H., Wensing, M.J.P., and Olde Rikkert, M.G.M. (2008) 'A randomised study of a multidisciplinary programme to intervene on geriatric syndromes in vulnerable older people who live at home (Dutch EASYcare Study)', *Journal of Gerontology Series A: Biological Sciences and Medical Sciences*, 63(3): 283–90.

Metzelthin, S., Rostgaard, T., Parsons, M. and Burton, E. (2020) 'Development of an internationally accepted definition of reablement: A Delphi study', *Ageing and Society*, 42(3): 703–18.

Moe, A., Ingstad, K., and Brataas, H.V. (2017) 'Patient influences in home-based reablement for older persons: qualitative research', *BMC Health Services Research*, 17(1): 736.

Netten, A., Ryan, M., Smith, P., Skatun, D., Healey, A., Knapp, M., and Wykes, T. (2002) 'The development of a measure of social care outcomes for older people', discussion paper 1690, Canterbury: University of Kent.

Newbronner, L., Baxter, M., Chamberlain, R., Maddison, J., Arksey, H., and Glendinning, C. (2007) 'Research into the longer term effects/impacts of re-ablement services', research report. London: Homecare Re-ablement Workstream, Care Services Efficiency Delivery Programme.

Parsons, J.G., Rose, P., Robinson, E., Sheridan, N., and Connolly, M. (2012) 'Goal setting as a feature of homecare services for older people: does it make a difference?', *Age and Ageing*, 41: 24–9.

Parsons, J.G., Sheridan, N., Rouse, N., Robinson E., and Connolly, M. (2013) 'A randomized controlled trial to determine the effect of a model of restorative home care on physical function and social support among older people', *Archives of Physical Medicine and Rehabilitation*, 94(6): 1015–22.

Parsons, M., Senior, H., Kerse, N., Chen, M., Jacobs, S., and Anderson, C. (2017) 'Randomised trial of restorative home care for frail older people in New Zealand', *Nursing Older People*, 29(7): 27–33.

Parsons, M., Parsons, J., Rouse, P., Pillai, A., Mathieson, S., Parsons, S., Smith, C., and Kenealy, T. (2018) 'Supported Discharge Teams for older people in hospital acute care: a randomised controlled trial', *Age and Ageing*, 47: 288–94.

Parsons, M., Parsons, J., Pillai, A., Rouse, P., Mathieson, S., Bregmen, R., Smith, C., and Kenealy, T. (2019) 'Post-acute care for older people following injury: a randomized controlled trial', *Journal of the American Medical Directors Association*, 21: 404–9.

Pettersson, C. and Iwarsson, S. (2017) 'Evidence-based interventions involving occupational therapists are needed in re-ablement for older community-living people: a systematic review', *British Journal of Occupational Therapy*, 80(5): 273–85.

Podsiadlo, D. and Richardson, S. (1991) 'The timed "Up and Go": a test of basic functional mobility for frail elderly persons', *Journal of American Geriatric Society*, 39: 142–8.

Reidy, H., Webber, M., Rayner, S., and Jones, M. (2013) *Evaluation of the Southwark Reablement Service*, London: Boroughs of Southwark, Croydon and Lewisham.

Rooijackers, T.H., Kempen, G., Zijlstra, G.A.R., van Rossum, E., Koster, A., Lima Passos, V., and Metzelthin, S. (2021) 'Effectiveness of a reablement training program for homecare staff on older adults' sedentary behavior: a cluster randomized controlled trial', *Journal of the American Geriatrics Society*, 69: 2566–78.

Ryburn, B., Wells, Y., and Foreman, P. (2009) 'Enabling independence: restorative approaches to home care provision for frail older adults', *Health & Social Care in the Community*, 17(3): 225–34.

Senior, H.E., Parsons, M., Kerse, N., Chen, M., Jacobs, S., Vander Hoorn, S., and Anderson, C.S. (2014) 'Promoting independence in frail older people: a randomised controlled trial of a restorative care service in New Zealand', *Age and Ageing*, 43(3): 418–24.

Sims-Gould, J., Tong, C.E., Wallis-Mayer, L., and Ashe, M.C. (2017) 'Reablement, reactivation, rehabilitation and restorative interventions with older adults in receipt of home care: a systematic review', *Journal of the American Medical Directors Association*, 18: 653–63.

Slater, P. and Hasson, F. (2018) 'An evaluation of the reablement service programme on physical ability, care needs and care plan packages', *Journal of Integrated Care*, 26(2): 140–9.

Szanton, S.L., Xue, Q.-L., Lef, B., Guralnik, J., Wolf, J.L., Tanner, E.K., Boyd, C., Thorpe, R.J., Bishai, D., and Gitlin, L.N. (2019) 'Effect of a biobehavioral environmental approach on disability among low-income older adults: a randomized clinical trial', *Journal of the American Medical Association Internal Medicine*, 179(2): 204–11.

Tessier, A., Beaulieu, M.D., McGinn, C.A., and Latulippe, R. (2016) 'Effectiveness of reablement: a systematic review', *Healthcare Policy*, 11(4): 49–59.

Tinetti, M., Baker, D., Gallo, W., Nanda, A., Charpentier, P., and O'Leary, J. (2002) 'Evaluation of restorative care vs usual care for older adults receiving an acute episode of home care', *Journal of the American Medical Association*, 287: 2098–105.

Tuntland, H., Aaslund, M.K., Espehaug, B., Førland, O., and Kjeken, I. (2015) 'Reablement in community-dwelling older adults: a randomised controlled trial', *BMC Geriatrics*, 15(143): 145.

University of Canberra Library (2022) 'Evidence-based practice in health' [online], Available from: https://canberra.libguides.com/c.php?g=599346&p=4149721.

Ware. Jr., J.E. and Sherbourne, C.D. (1992) 'The MOS 36–item short-form health survey (SF-36): I. Conceptual framework and item selection', *Medical Care*, 30(6): 473–83.

Whitehead, P.J., Worthington, E.J., Parry, R.H., Walker, M.F., and Drummond, A.E.R. (2015) 'Interventions to reduce dependency in personal activities of daily living in community dwelling adults who use homecare services: a systematic review', *Clinical Rehabilitation*, 29(11): 1064–76.

Whitehead, P.J., Walker, M.F., Parry, R.H., Latif, Z., McGeorge, I.D., and Drummond, A.E.R. (2016) 'Occupational Therapy in HomEcare Reablement Services (OTHERS): results of a feasibility randomised controlled trial', *BMJ Open*, 6(8): e011868.

Wilde, A. and Glendinning, C. (2012) 'If they're helping me then how can I be independent? The perceptions and experience of users of home-care re-ablement services', *Health & Social Care in the Community*, 20(6): 583–90.

Winkel, A., Langberg, H., and Wæhrens, E.E. (2015) 'Reablement in a community setting', *Disability and Rehabilitation*, 37(15): 1347–52.

Zingmark, M. and Bernspång, B. (2011) 'Meeting the needs of elderly with bathing disability', *Australian Occupational Therapy Journal*, 58: 164–71.

6

Examining client-level outcomes and instruments in reablement

Hanne Tuntland, Daniel Doh, Maria Ranner, Susanne Guidetti,
and Magnus Zingmark

Introduction

Given the interdisciplinary nature of reablement, the various components the intervention consists of, and the wide range of potential outcomes needed to evaluate the effects of reablement, there is clearly a need to elaborate the issue of client-level outcomes within the context of reablement. As presented also in the previous chapter, the term *client-level outcomes* refers to outcomes that are directly associated with the individual who is engaged in reablement, such as increased mobility or quality of life. Ideally, there is a logical link between what the intervention intends to affect and the outcome measure that is used to evaluate that effect (Whyte and Hart, 2003; Coster, 2013). Thus, there is a need for a good match between the outcomes that reablement (per definition) is intended to affect and the instruments that are used to capture these outcomes (Coster, 2013).

In this chapter, the issue of client-level outcomes for evaluating reablement is elaborated. The chapter examines client-level outcomes and instruments used in empirical, clinical trials regarding reablement, and provides an overview of this. In clinical practice and research, outcomes are used to identify changes in the client's health condition and functioning over time. The chapter is not about what clients have identified as their preferred outcomes, but rather what the researchers of the included studies have identified as relevant outcomes. The chapter presents what outcomes and instruments have been applied in the reablement research, as there is a lack of such an overview in the existing literature. There has been a tendency for some reablement researchers, in particular within the Scandinavian countries, to be inspired by each other to use the same outcomes and instruments as used in earlier published studies, possibly without a comprehensive understanding of what outcomes and instruments would be preferable to use. Nonetheless, the authors of this chapter hypothesise that there is a wide range of outcomes and instruments being used, and little consistency across studies and countries globally, which is hampering comparability (see also

Chapter 5 by Lewin et al). Hence, the chapter investigates which client-level outcomes and instruments to measure client-level outcomes have been used in clinical trials in various countries. Based on the findings, the chapter also includes recommendations with regards to which outcomes might be used in clinical practice and research.

Methods

The chapter uses a literature review and comparative cluster analysis to examine which client-level outcomes and measurement instruments have been applied in reablement interventions in different studies across the world. The inclusion criteria for the selected papers were based on: 1. the reablement literature concurred with the definition of reablement (Metzelthin et al, 2020); 2. research literature from 2010 and onwards; 3. planned or conducted clinical trials published in peer-reviewed journals; and 4. trials published in the English language. If several publications dealt with the same trial, only one publication was chosen. The literature search was conducted with assistance from a librarian in MEDLINE, EMBASE and CINAHL databases using the English terms *reablement*, *re-ablement* and *restorative care* as search terms, and was completed in June 2021. The focus was on empirical and clinical trials to examine what has been used in the reablement intervention research literature. The clinical trials were of various study designs, such as randomised controlled trials, clinical controlled trials, and cohort studies. Although complying with the definition of reablement, studies deriving from institutional care such as nursing homes were excluded. As this chapter is not a systematic review of effectiveness studies, the intention was not to exhaustively include all relevant effectiveness studies within reablement, but to analyse some trends in outcomes for clients and measurement instruments used across a collection of empirical studies.

Findings

The current analysis comprised 18 research papers from nine countries – Australia (5), New Zealand (5), Norway (2), Denmark (1), Japan (1), Sweden (1), Taiwan (1), the Netherlands (1), and the United Kingdom (1). The analysis considers the specific client-level outcomes that have been presented in the studies and the measurement instruments that were used. Table 6.1 provides an overview of all studies included.

Client-level outcomes

Table 6.2 summarises the client-level outcomes and the number of times they were used across the included studies, demonstrating the diversity

Table 6.1: Client-level outcomes and measurement instruments in reablement studies

Source country	Authors/year	Study design	Client-level outcomes	Measurement instruments
Australia	Burton et al, 2013	A randomised controlled trial	Static balance	Functional reach
			Strength	Chair sit to stand one and five times
			Functional mobility	Timed Up and Go (TUG)
			Dynamic balance	Tandem walk
			Confidence regarding completing more challenging tasks without falling	Falls Efficacy Scale Activities-specific Balance Confidence scale
			Effect on pain levels, sleep, appetite, and mental and physical wellbeing	Vitality plus scale
			Level of function and disability in everyday activities	Late life function and disability instruments
Australia	Burton et al, 2014	A randomised controlled trial	Maintaining upright posture	Functional reach
			Chair stand performance	Chair sit to stand
			Functional mobility	Timed Up and Go (TUG)
			Gait	Tandem walk
			Confidence, fear of falling	Falls Efficacy Scale
			Confidence, activity-related balance	Activities-specific Balance Confidence scale
			Health-related benefits of exercise	Vitality plus scale
			Functional limitations and disability	Late life function and disability instruments
Australia	Jeon et al, 2019	Study protocol for a randomised controlled trial and realist evaluation	Functional independence (self-care disability and independent living skills)	Disability Assessment for Dementia (DAD)

Table 6.1: Client-level outcomes and measurement instruments in reablement studies (continued)

Source country	Authors/year	Study design	Client-level outcomes	Measurement instruments
			Physical function	Short Physical Performance Battery (SPPB)
			Depression	Geriatric Depression Scale: 15-item (CS-GDS-15)
			Quality of life	Quality of life in Alzheimer's disease (QOL-AD)
			Health related quality of life	The European Quality of Life Scale (EQ-5D-5L)
			Falls	*
Australia	Lewin and Vandermeulen, 2010	A clinical controlled trial	Functional independence in ADL	Activities of Daily Living (ADL) scales based on the modified Barthel index
			Functional independence in IADL	Instrumental Activities of Daily Living (IADL) scale based on the Lawton and Brody scale
			Mobility/balance	Timed Up and Go (TUG)
			Confidence	The Modified Falls Efficacy Scale (MFES)
			Wellbeing	Philadelphia Geriatric Morale Scale (PGMS)
Australia	Lewin et al, 2013	A randomised controlled trial	Functional independence in ADL	Activities of Daily Living (ADL) scales based on the modified Barthel index
			Functional independence in IADL	Instrumental Activities of Daily Living (IADL) scale based on the Lawton and Brody scale

(continued)

Table 6.1: Client-level outcomes and measurement instruments in reablement studies (continued)

Source country	Authors/year	Study design	Client-level outcomes	Measurement instruments
			Mobility/balance	Timed Up and Go (TUG)
			Confidence	Modified Falls Efficacy Scale (MFES)
			Quality of life	Assessment of Quality of Life (AQOL) scale
Denmark	Winkel et al, 2015	A cohort study	ADL ability	ADL-interview (ADL-I), ADL taxonomy
Japan	Hattori et al, 2019	A randomised controlled trial	Independence from long-term care services	Administrative claims data and interviews with care managers*
			Serious adverse events	*
The Netherlands	Rooijackers et al, 2021	A randomised controlled trial	Sedentary time	Tri-axial wrist-worn accelerometer
			Daily functioning in (I)ADL	Groningen Activity Restriction Scale (GARS)
			Physical functioning	Short Physical Performance Battery (SPPB)
			Psychological functioning	The Patient Health Questionnaire – 9 (PHQ-9)
			Falls	Registration of number of falls during last 6 months*
New Zealand	King et al, 2012	A randomised controlled trial	Health-related quality of life	Short Form 36 (SF36) Health Survey
			Functional mobility	Nottingham Extended Activities of Daily Living (NEADL)
			Mobility	Timed Up and Go (TUG)
			Sense of control	Mastery scale

Table 6.1: Client-level outcomes and measurement instruments in reablement studies (continued)

Source country	Authors/year	Study design	Client-level outcomes	Measurement instruments
			Social support network	Duke Social Support Index (DSSI)
New Zealand	Parsons and Parsons, 2012	A randomised controlled trial	Successful identification of a goal in the client's clinical record	*Clinical record
			Functional independence in EADL	Nottingham Extended Activities of Daily Living (NEADL)
			Functional independence in ADL	Barthel Scale
			Quality of life	EQ-5D
			Cognitive state	Abbreviated Mental Test Score
New Zealand	Parsons et al, 2013	A randomised controlled trial	Physical functions	Short Physical Performance Battery (SPPB)
			Social support	Duke Social Support Index (DSSI)
New Zealand	Parsons et al, 2017	A randomised controlled trial	Death or permanent institutional care	*
			Functional ability: ADL, IADL, Cognitive, Depression, and Pain	Inter-RAI Home Care (physical function, health, social support, and service use)
			Current health status	EuroQoL thermometer visual analogue scale
New Zealand	Senior et al, 2014	A randomised controlled trial	Death	The Regional health office mortality*
			Performance in ADL, performance in IADL, pain perception, cognitive performance, severity of depression, instability in health	Inter-RAI home care (interRAI-HC, ver 2.03)
			Current health status	EQ-5D

(continued)

Table 6.1: Client-level outcomes and measurement instruments in reablement studies (continued)

Source country	Authors/year	Study design	Client-level outcomes	Measurement instruments
			Adverse events (AEs)	Adverse events (AEs) and serious AEs were systematically monitored and reported*
Norway	Langeland et al, 2019	A clinical controlled trial	Performance of daily activities and satisfaction with that performance	Canadian Occupational Performance Measure (COPM)
			Physical function	Short Physical Performance Battery (SPPB)
			Health-related quality of life	The European Quality of Life Scale (EQ-5D-5L)
			Coping related to experience of coherence in life	The Sense of Coherence questionnaire (SOC-13)
Norway	Tuntland et al, 2015	A randomised controlled trial	Performance of daily activities and satisfaction with that performance	Canadian Occupational Performance Measure (COPM)
			Functional mobility	Timed Up and Go (TUG)
			Grip strength	Jamar dynamometer
			Health-related quality of life	COOP/Wonka
Sweden	Bergström et al, 2019	A study protocol for a feasibility study (cohort study)	Self-assessed performance and satisfaction of valued activities in everyday life	Canadian Occupational Performance Measure (COPM)
			Dependence/ independence of assistance in ADL	Barthel/Katz extended activities of daily living (ADL)
			Participation of performing social activities and everyday activities	Frenchay Activity Index (FAI)

Table 6.1: Client-level outcomes and measurement instruments in reablement studies (continued)

Source country	Authors/year	Study design	Client-level outcomes	Measurement instruments
			Perceived belief in one's ability in different situations	General Self-Efficacy (GSE) scale
			Health-related quality of life	EQ-5D
			Anxiety and depression	Hospital Anxiety and Depression (HAD) scale
			Emotional-, social-, and psychological wellbeing	Mental Health Continuum: Short Form, Swedish version (MHC-SF)
			Community integration	Reintegration to Normal Living (RNL)
			Sense of health (salutogenesis)	Sense of coherence (short form)
			Falls	*
Taiwan	Chiang et al, 2020	A clinical controlled trial	Disability level (self-care difficulty)	Barthel Index
			Health related quality of life	WHO quality of life-BREF
United Kingdom	Beresford et al, 2019	A cohort study	Health related quality of life	EQ-5D-5L
			Social care-related quality of life	Adult Social Care Outcomes Toolkit (ASCOT SCT-4)
			Self-report measure of current mental health	General Health Questionnaire
			Functional status of daily living and personal grooming	Barthel activities of daily living index
			A self-report measure of functional ability	Nottingham Extended ADL scale

Note: * These are not measurement instruments, but other kinds for registration of outcomes.

Table 6.2: Unique client-level outcomes

Client-level outcomes	Subcategory of included outcome	Number of times used across the included studies
Functional independence in ADL	• Functional independence in ADL • Functional independence in IADL • Functional independence in EADL • Functional independence (Self-care disability and independent living skills) • Performance in ADL • Performance in IADL • Performance of daily activities • Daily functioning in (I)ADL • ADL ability • Level of function and disability in everyday activities • Independence from long-term care services • Dependence/independence of assistance in ADL • Participation of performing social activities and everyday activities • Functional status of daily living and personal grooming • A self-report measure of functional ability • Disability level (self-care difficulty)	23
Physical functioning	• Mobility/balance • Functional mobility • Chair stand performance • Gait • Maintaining upright posture • Physical function • Falls • Functional limitations and disability • Mobility • Physical capacity, functional mobility • Grip strength • Static balance • Strength • Dynamic balance	22
Health-related quality of life	• Health-related quality of life • Wellbeing • Quality of life • Health-related benefits of exercise • Health-related quality of life • Sense of health (salutogenesis) • Social care-related quality of life • Current health status • Instability in health	17

Table 6.2: Unique client-level outcomes (continued)

Client-level outcomes	Subcategory of included outcome	Number of times used across the included studies
Psychological functioning	• Psychological functioning • Cognitive state • Social support • Social support network • Coping related to experience of coherence in life • Effect on pain levels, sleep, appetite, and mental and physical wellbeing • Anxiety and depression • Depression • Cognitive performance • Emotional-, social-, and psychological wellbeing • Self-report measure of current mental health • Pain	16
Confidence	• Confidence • Confidence – fear of falling • Confidence-activity-related balance • Confidence regarding completing more challenging tasks without falling • Perceived belief in one's ability in different situations	6
Satisfaction of performance of ADL	• Satisfaction of performance of ADL	3
Adverse events (AEs)	• Serious adverse events	2
Death	• Death • Death or permanent institutional care	2
Sedentary behaviour	• Sedentary time	
Sense of control		1
Social participation	• Community integration	1
Successful identification of a goal in the client's clinical record		1

of client-level outcomes. The outcomes are clustered into 12 reablement outcomes across the 18 studies. The outcomes include functional independence in ADL, physical function, health-related quality of life, psychological functioning, confidence, satisfaction of performance of ADL, adverse events, death, sedentary behaviour, sense of control, social participation, and successful identification of a goal in clients' clinical record.

Table 6.3: Measurement instruments used for client-level outcomes

Measurement instruments (41)	Number of times the instruments are used across the included studies
Barthel ADL Index	6
European Quality of Life Scale (EQ-5D and EQ-5D-5L)	6
Timed Up and Go	6
Falls Efficacy Scale and Modified Falls Efficacy Scale (MFES) (Confident)	4
Short Physical Performance Battery (SPPB)	4
Canadian Occupational Performance Measure (COPM)	3
Nottingham Extended Activities of Daily Living (NEADL)	3
Duke Social Support Index (DSSI)	2
Instrumental Activities of Daily Living (IADL) scale (Lawton and Brody scale)	2
Inter-RAI home care	2
Tandem walk	2
Functional reach	2
Chair sit to stand	2
Sense of Coherence questionnaire (SOC-13)	2
Late life function and disability instruments	2
Vitality plus scale	2
Activities-specific Balance Confidence (ABC) scale	2
Short Form 36 (SF36) Health Survey	1
Philadelphia Geriatric Morale Scale (PGMS)	1
Jamar dynamometer	1
Mastery scale	1
COOP/Wonka	1
Assessment of Quality of Life (AQOL) scale	1
WHO quality of life-BREF	1
Abbreviated Mental Test Score	1
ADL-interview (ADL-I), ADL taxonomy	1
Tri-axial wrist-worn accelerometer	1
Groningen Activity Restriction Scale (GARS)	1
Frenchay Activity Index (FAI)	1
General Self-Efficacy (GSE) scale	1

Table 6.3: Measurement instruments used for client-level outcomes (continued)

Measurement instruments (41)	Number of times the instruments are used across the included studies
Hospital Anxiety and Depression (HAD) scale	1
Geriatric Depression Scale: 15-item (CS-GDS-15)	1
The Patient Health Questionnaire – 9 (PHQ-9)	1
Mental Health Continuum: Short Form, Swedish version (MHC-SF)	1
Reintegration to Normal Living (RNL)	1
Adult Social Care Outcomes Toolkit (ASCOT SCT-4)	1
General Health Questionnaire	1
Disability Assessment for Dementia (DAD)	1
Quality of life in Alzheimer's disease (QOL-AD)	1
EuroQoL thermometer visual analogue scale	1
Katz extended scale	1

Functional independence, which comprises activities of daily living, was the most frequently used client outcome across the studies. All countries except Japan have used this outcome. It is important to acknowledge that while most of the literature focused on managing activities of daily living (ADL), there is a need to provide further explanation of the term and other related concepts, which in the analysis were clustered to form the outcome functional independence in ADL. The term ADL is in this chapter used as an umbrella term referring to the kind of activities undertaken purposely to promote everyday living. The term is also used for activities that are oriented toward taking care of your own body, often termed PADL (Personal Activities of Daily Living). The term IADL (Instrumental Activities of Daily Living) refers to activities that support daily life, are oriented toward interacting with your environment, whereas the term EADL (Extended Activities of Daily Living) refers to activities beyond self-care and are necessary for independent living.

The second most frequently used client-level outcome across the included studies is *physical functioning*. The physical functioning outcome includes subcategories such as mobility, posture, disability, grip, walking, strength, and getting up. This outcome was seen mostly in studies from Australia, the Netherlands, New Zealand, and Norway.

The third most used client-level outcome was *health-related quality of life*, while *psychological functioning* came as number four. Health-related quality of life comprises wellbeing, quality of life, health and functioning. Most studies from New Zealand, Norway, Taiwan, and

United Kingdom captured these outcomes. Psychological functioning comprises subcategories such as cognition, depression, experiences of coherence in life and social support. These outcomes are captured in studies from Australia, the Netherlands, New Zealand, Norway, Sweden, and United Kingdom.

Measurement instruments

Proceeding to look into how the client-level outcomes were measured in various instruments, Table 6.3 shows the measurement instruments used in determining client-level outcomes in reablement interventions. Overall, there were 41 instruments being used across 1 to 6 of the studies included. From the cluster analysis, three instruments were most pronounced in reablement measurement: Barthel ADL Index (Mahoney and Barthel, 1965), European Quality of Life Scale (EQ-5D-5L) (Euroqol-group, 1990), and Timed Up and Go (TUG) (Podsiadlo and Richardson, 1991). The ADL measurements were mostly used in studies in Australia, Denmark, New Zealand, Norway, Sweden, and the United Kingdom. Besides the Barthel ADL Index, the Canadian Occupational Performance Measure (COPM) (Law et al, 2015), the Nottingham Extended Activities of Daily Living (NEADL) (Nouri and Lincoln, 1987), the Instrumental Activities of Daily Living (IADL) scale (Lawton and Brody scale) (Lawton and Brody, 1969), and the inter-RAI Home Care (Landi et al, 2000), are examples of instruments used to capture activities of daily living.

The European Quality of Life Scale (EQ-5D-5L) was also much used across studies in Australia, New Zealand, Norway, Sweden, and United Kingdom. However, some studies only used the visual analogue scale to identify the current health status. Hence, not all included the five domains nor the five-level version of each domain. In addition, the Short Form 36 (SF36) Health Survey (Ware and Sherbourne, 1992) was used in New Zealand to measure health-related quality of life. The Timed Up and Go (TUG), which was used to measure functional mobility skills, featured prominently in studies in Australia, New Zealand, and Norway. However, the Short Physical Performance Battery (SPPB) (Guralnik et al, 1994) was also used to measure physical function/mobility.

Other significant measurements of client-level outcomes in reablement interventions according to the analysis in Table 6.3 were the Falls Efficacy Scale (Tinetti et al, 1990) and Modified Falls Efficacy Scale (MFES) (Confident) (Hill et al, 1996). These instruments were mostly used in studies in Australia. The analysis further demonstrates there is significant variability in measuring client-level outcomes in reablement studies across the included studies as 41 measurements were identified.

Discussion

This chapter has identified which client-level outcomes and instruments have been used in clinical trials in various countries. In clinical practice, understanding and measuring client-level outcomes in reablement is critical in care arrangements for people who need support to live meaningful lives. The findings also show that there is a great variety of outcomes and instruments used in empirical research, a finding that is supported in a systematic review assessing instruments used to measure ADL functioning (Buma et al, 2022). The initial assumption that there is a wide range of outcomes and instruments being used and little consistency across studies and countries proved to be correct. However, the inconsistency across countries is hampering the comparability of results between countries and studies, as also emphasised in Chapter 5 by Lewin et al. More importantly, it is also hindering meta-analyses to be conducted and as a result providing limited evidence for the effectiveness of reablement.

The studies included in this chapter cover research on reablement from nine countries. One of the most often measured client-level outcomes is functional independence in activities of daily living. In addition, physical functioning, psychological functioning, and health-related quality of life outcomes were commonly used. In total, 41 instruments were used across the various studies. The findings are consistent with the conclusions in Chapter 10 by Clothworthy and Westendorp and previous research (Doh et al, 2019) indicating that the main focus of reablement services has been on ADL and physical function, whereas needs related to leisure and social participation have often remained unmet. Taken together, and beyond the findings in our chapter, there is a clear need to also consider client-level outcomes addressing a broader scope, in particular including social connectedness (Nyman et al, 2014).

According to the Delphi definition, reablement 'aims to enhance an individual's physical and/or other functioning and to increase or maintain their independence in meaningful activities of daily living' (Metzelthin et al, 2020: 713). Hence, the client-level outcomes that reablement aims to improve are physical functioning, other functioning, and performance in meaningful activities. The outcome 'other functioning' is not specified in the definition, but could presumably include both psychological, cognitive, and social functioning. Tables 6.2 and 6.3 show that the most frequently used outcomes and instruments are those who are measuring functional outcomes such as ADL, physical functioning, and psychological functioning. This confirms that there is a logical link between how reablement intends to affect client outcomes and the instruments used to capture that outcome, as recommended by Coster (2013). However, there appears to be one mismatch. Health-related quality of life is not specified in the definition as an outcome to improve, but it is nonetheless much used as an outcome in the included trials. Yet functional independence in ADL, physical functioning, psychological functioning, and social functioning are important dimensions of many QQL instruments, such as European Quality of Life Scale (EQ-5D), Short Form (SF36), Adult Social Care Outcomes Toolkit (ASCOT SCT-4) and COOP/Wonka. Therefore, it could be stated that health-related quality of life could potentially be seen as a functional outcome.

Selecting appropriate instruments can be challenging. Relevant questions to ask are: what outcomes are important to measure, to what degree does a specific instrument provide a valid and reliable assessment, and is the selected instrument able to capture true changes over time (Kjeken, 2012). However, this selection process may not have been conducted ideally in the included studies leading to the great variety of outcomes and instruments being used. One reason for this is that researchers tend to use instruments they already are familiar with. Another reason is that it varies which instruments are translated from the original language (often English) to the language of the research team. As translation and cultural adaptation of an instrument is time-consuming and require methodological expertise (Wild et al, 2005), researchers tend to use instruments that already exist in their respective languages. In addition, sound psychometric properties may not have received sufficient consideration due to the lack of translated instruments. Moreover, given the rehabilitative intervention is still in its infancy, it is unknown to what extent the intervention could improve certain outcomes. There might, to a certain degree, have been conducted a trial-and-error exercise when selecting relevant instruments.

Finally, some conclusions regarding a core set of client-level outcomes and measurements. Having a recommended core set of client-level outcomes and instruments would promote the use of suitable outcomes and instruments, enhance the translation of instruments, and provide comparable data to be used in meta-analysis. A suggested core set for instruments used in reablement to measure client-level outcomes should include both subjective and objective measures. This core set of outcomes and measurements should cover client-level outcomes of performance in daily activities/ADL, physical functioning, and health-related quality of life. Since the psychometric properties of the instruments included in this chapter have not been evaluated, it is outside the scope of the chapter to prescribe instruments for capturing client-level outcomes.

Limitations

As this chapter is not a systematic review, the intention was not to exhaustively include all empirical reablement studies globally. Hence, a comprehensive literature search was not conducted. As a result, relevant studies may not have been identified for inclusion.

The suggestions for a core set of outcomes must be regarded as tentative. To provide a stronger recommendation for a core set of outcomes and instruments used in reablement, psychometric properties should be assessed, and a Delphi study should be conducted.

Conclusion

In this chapter, an analysis of 18 studies from nine countries including Australia, Denmark, Japan, the Netherlands, New Zealand, Norway, Sweden, Taiwan, and the United Kingdom has been conducted. In all, 12 categories of client-level outcomes were identified. Functional independence in ADL, physical functioning and health-related quality of life were the most frequently used outcomes. In all, a total of 41 instruments were used, of which the Barthel ADL Index, European Quality of Life Scale (EQ-5D), and Timed Up and Go (TUG) were the ones most frequently used.

Given the lack of consistency regarding client-level outcomes and instruments used in reablement research, a set of core outcomes and instruments would enhance comparison between studies and stronger evidence in meta-analysis. A core set of outcomes should as a minimum cover the client-level outcomes of performance in daily activities/ADL, physical functioning, and health-related quality of life. In addition, there is also a need to consider client-level outcomes addressing social connectedness.

Acknowledgements
We thank Rudi Westendorp and Sasmita Kusumastuti for their contributions on an early stage of this chapter.

References
Beresford, B., Mayhew, E., Duarte, A., Faria, R., Weatherly, H., Mann, R., Parker, G., Aspinal, F., and Kanaan, M. (2019) 'Outcomes of reablement and their measurement: Findings from an evaluation of English reablement services', *Health & Social Care in the Community*, 27(6): 1438–50.

Bergström, A., Borell, L., Meijer, S., and Guidetti, S. (2019) 'Evaluation of an intervention addressing a reablement programme for older, community-dwelling persons in Sweden (ASSIST 1.0): a protocol for a feasibility study', *BMJ Open*, 9(7): e025870.

Buma, L., Vluggen, S., Zwakhalen, S., Kempen, I.J.M., and Methzelthin, S. (2022) 'Effects on clients' daily functioning and common features of reablement interventions: a systematic literature review', *European Journal of Ageing*. DOI: 10.1007/s10433-022-000693-3

Burton, E., Lewin, G., Clemson, L., and Boldy, D. (2013) 'Effectiveness of a lifestyle exercise program for older people receiving a restorative home care service: a pragmatic randomized controlled trial', *Clinical Intervention in Aging*, 8: 1591–601.

Burton, E., Lewin, G., Clemson, L., and Boldy, D. (2014) 'Long-term benefits of a lifestyle exercise program for older people receiving a restorative home care service: a pragmatic randomized controlled trial', *Healthy Aging & Clinical Care in the Elderly*, 6: 1–9.

Chiang, Y.H., Hsu, H.C., Chen, C.L., Chen, C.F., Chang-Lee, S.N., Chen, Y.M., and Hsu, S.W. (2020) 'Evaluation of reablement home care: effects on care attendants, care recipients, and family caregivers', *International Journal of Environmental Research and Public Health*, 17(23): 8784.

Coster, W.J. (2013) 'Making the best match: selecting outcome measures for clinical trials and outcome studies', *American Journal of Occupational Therapy*, 67(2): 162–70.

Doh, D., Smith, R., and Gevers, P. (2019) 'Reviewing the reablement approach to caring for older people', *Ageing & Society*, 40(6): 1371–83.

EuroQol-group (1990) 'EuroQol – a facility for the measurement of health-related quality of life', *Health Policy*, 16: 199–208.

Francis, J., Fisher, M., and Rutter D. (2011) 'Reablement: a cost-effective route to better outcomes', Research Briefing 36, London: Social Care Institute for Excellence.

Guralnik, J., Simonsick, E., and Ferruci, K. (1994) 'A short physical performance battery assessing lower extremity function: association with self-reported disability and prediction of mortality and nursing home admission', *Journal of Gerontology*, 49(2): M85–94.

Hattori, S., Yoshira, T., Okumura, Y., and Kondo, K. (2019) 'Effects of reablement on the independence of community-dwelling older adults with mild disability: a randomized controlled trial', *International Journal of Environmental Research and Public Health*, 16: 3954.

Hill, K.D., Schwarz, J.A., Kalogeropoulos, A.J., and Gibson, S.J. (1996) 'Fear of falling revisited', *Archives of Physical Medicine and Rehabilitation*, 77(10): 1025–9.

Jeon, Y.-H., Simpson, J.M., Low, L.-F., Woods, R., Norman, R., Mowszowski, L., Clemson, L., Naismith, S.L., Brodaty, H., and Hilmer, S. (2019) 'A pragmatic randomised controlled trial (RCT) and realist evaluation of the interdisciplinary home-bAsed Reablement program (I-HARP) for improving functional independence of community dwelling older people with dementia: an effectiveness-implementation hybrid design', *BMC Geriatrics*, 19(1): 199.

King, A.I., Parsons, M., Robinson, E., and Jorgensen, D. (2012) 'Assessing the impact of a restorative home care service in New Zealand: a cluster randomised controlled trial', *Health & Social Care in the Community*, 20(4): 365–74.

Kjeken I. (2012) 'Measurement in occupational therapy', *Scandinavian Journal of Occupational Therapy*, 19(6): 466–7.

Landi, F., Tua, E., Onder, G., Carrara, B., Sgadari, A., Rinaldi, C., Gambassi, G., Lattanzio, F., and Bernabei, R. (2000) 'Minimum data set for home care: a valid instrument to assess frail older people living in the community', *Medical Care*, 1184–90.

Langeland, E., Tuntland, H., Folkestad, B., Førland, O., Jacobsen, F., and Kjeken, I. (2019) 'A multicenter investigation of reablement in Norway: a clinical controlled trial', *BMC Geriatrics*, 19(29).

Law, M., Baptiste, S., Carswell, A., McColl, M., Polatajko, H., and Pollock, N. (2015) *COPM Canadian Occupational Performance Measure (Norwegian version)*, Oslo: NKRR National advisory unit on rehabilitation in rheumatology.

Lawton, M.P. and Brody, E.M. (1969) 'Assessment of older people: self-maintaining and instrumental activities of daily living', *The Gerontologist*, 9(3, Part 1): 179–86.

Lewin, G. and Vandermeulen, S. (2010) 'A non-randomised controlled trial of the Home Independence Program (HIP): an Australian restorative programme for older home-care clients', *Health & Social Care in the Community*, 18(1): 91–9.

Lewin, G., De San Miguel, K., Knuiman, M., Alan, J., Boldy, D., and Hendrie, D. (2013) 'A randomised controlled trial of the Home Independence Program, an Australian restorative home-care programme for older adults', *Health & Social Care in the Community*, 21(Jan): 69–78.

Mahoney, F.I. and Barthel, D.W. (1965) 'Functional evaluation. The Barthel Index: a simple index of independence useful in scoring improvement in the rehabilitation of the chronically ill', *Maryland State Medical Journal*, 14:61–5.

Metzelthin, S., Rostgaard, T., Parsons, M., and Burton, E. (2020) 'Development of an internationally accepted definition of reablement: a Delphi study', *Ageing and Society*, 42(3): 703–18.

Nouri, F. and Lincoln, N. (1987) 'An extended activities of daily living scale for stroke patients', *Clinical Rehabilitation*, 1(4): 301–5.

Nyman, A., Josephsson, S., and Isaksson, G. (2014) 'Being part of an unfolding story: togetherness in everyday occupations when ageing', *Scandinavian Journal of Occupational Therapy*, 21(5): 368–76.

Parsons, J.G.M. and Parsons, M.J.G. (2012) 'The effect of a designated tool on person-centred goal identification and service planning among older people receiving homecare in New Zealand', *Health & Social Care in the Community*, 20(6): 653–62.

Parsons, J.G.M., Sheridan, N., Rouse, P., Robinson, E., and Connolly, M. (2013) 'A randomized controlled trial to determine the effect of a model of restorative home care on physical function and social support among older people', *Archives of Physical Medicine Rehabilitation*, 94(6): 1015–22.

Parsons, M., Senior, H., Kerse, N., Chen, M.H., Jacobs, S., and Anderson, C. (2017) 'Randomised trial of restorative home care for frail older people in New Zealand', *Nursing Older People*, 29(7): 27–33.

Podsiadlo, D. and Richardson, S. (1991) 'The timed "Up & Go": a test of basic functional mobility for frail elderly persons', *Journal of American Geriatric Society*, 39(2): 142–8.

Rooijackers, T., Kempen, G.I., Zijlstra, G.R., van Rossum, E., Koster, A., Passos, V.L., and Metzelthin, S. (2021) 'Effectiveness of a reablement training program on self-efficacy and outcome expectations regarding client activation in homecare staff: a cluster randomized controlled trial', *Journal of the American Geriatrics Society*, 69(9): 2566–78.

Senior, H.E., Parsons, M., Kerse, N., Chen, M., Jacobs, S., and Anderson, C. (2014) 'Promoting independence in frail older people: a randomised controlled trial of a restorative care service in New Zealand', *Age & Ageing*, 43(3): 418–24.

Tinetti, M.E., Richman, D., and Powell, L. (1990) 'Falls efficacy as a measure of fear of falling', *Journal of Gerontology*, 45(6): P239–43.

Tuntland, H., Aaslund, M., Espehaug, B., Førland, O., and Kjeken, I. (2015) 'Reablement in community-dwelling older adults: a randomised controlled trial', *BMC Geriatrics*, 15(146): 1–11.

Ware, J.J. and Sherbourne, C. (1992) 'The MOS 36-item short-form health survey (SF-36): I. Conceptual framework and item selection', *Medical Care*, 30(6): 473–83.

Whyte, J. and Hart, T. (2003) 'It's more than a black box; it's a Russian doll: defining rehabilitation treatments', *American Journal of Physical Medicine and Rehabilitation*, 82(8): 639–52.

Wild, D., Grove, A., Martin, M., Eremenco, S., McElroy, S., Verjee-Lorenz, A., and Erikson, P. (2005) 'Principles of good practice for the translation and cultural adaptation process for patient-reported outcomes (PRO) measures: report of the ISPOR Task Force for Translation and Cultural Adaptation', *Value in Health*, 8(2): 94–104.

Winkel, A., Langberg, H., and Wæhrens, E.E. (2015) 'Reablement in a community setting', *Disability and Rehabilitation*, 37(15): 1347–52.

7

Reablement as a cost-effective option from a health economic perspective

Magnus Zingmark, Hanne Tuntland, and Elissa Burton

Introduction

Reablement has been seen as an answer to a number of enduring challenges in long-term care for older people, including a means to promote health among older people as well as to reduce the societal costs related to a fast-growing older population (Aspinal et al, 2016). Reablement has the potential to be a cost-effective option when resources need to be prioritised in health and social care. In any organisation, or health and social care system, resources are scarce; consequently, choices need to be made concerning which interventions to implement. When considering whether to implement reablement as an alternative to compensatory home care, the choice must also take into account what it costs and whether it is more costly than the usual approach, given the results that it may produce.

Health economic methods can guide such choices by considering both the effects of different interventions and their related costs (Drummond et al, 2005). Ultimately, a health economic evaluation can guide clinicians as well as decision-makers on which intervention yields the most health benefits given the existing resources. Therefore, in order to reflect over the existing evidence base, identify knowledge gaps and to guide policy making and future research, it is important to summarise the health economic literature and look into what it may teach us on the cost-effectiveness of reablement.

Following an introduction to health economic evaluation methods, the aim of this chapter is to provide a summary of existing evidence on the cost-effectiveness of reablement, based on a brief literature review, and to discuss health economic perspectives of reablement from a clinical and future research perspective.

Health economic evaluation methods

Health economic evaluation refers to a set of methods that can be used to identify the most efficient use of resources by considering both health effects and costs (Drummond et al, 2005). In relation to any intervention, a cost-analysis can be conducted, that is, to evaluate which costs are involved in the delivery of an intervention, as well as how other costs are affected by the intervention. With regards to reablement, the costs for the reablement period can be considered the intervention costs whereas savings related to reduced need for home care or special housing could be considered 'other costs'. However, both costs and effects need to be considered for a full economic evaluation. In the following sections, different methods and their main characteristics are described in short.

Cost-minimisation and cost-analysis

When two interventions result in the same effect on the health outcome evaluated (such as improved independence in carrying out daily activities) and the only difference is the cost, a cost-minimisation analysis can be undertaken. Thus, how the cost is identified, measured, and valued is a critical feature that needs to be clearly described. Therefore, the next section also applies to all other types of health economic evaluations.

A range of costs can be included for analysis such as (a) direct costs related to the provision of the intervention; (b) other health and/or social care related costs (that is admission to hospital, home care use, medications); (c) private costs (that is transportation, equipment); and (d) productivity, (that is, the value of formal or informal work or caregiving). Precisely which costs are to be included depends on the perspective from which the health economic evaluation is conducted. The general recommendation in health economic evaluation is to apply a societal perspective, including all costs such as healthcare, social care, and informal care (Drummond et al, 2005). The central argument for this recommendation is that decision-making needs to consider all relevant costs and effects of interventions independent of in which sector they occur. However, a service provider perspective can also be applied, in which only some costs particular for this provider are included. Taking the service model applied in Sweden as an example, from a municipality perspective, the cost for the intervention and home care would be relevant since these costs are financed by the municipality, whereas hospital costs would be less relevant since they are financed by the region. In addition, in relation to the direct costs identified, other features that are important to consider are how costs are measured and valued and for how long time costs are followed.

Cost-effectiveness and cost-utility analysis

Cost-effectiveness analysis is the most common form of health economic evaluation used in the health sector. In cost-effectiveness analysis, costs and effects of two or more interventions are compared, and the evaluation includes an effect in terms of a health outcome (Drummond et al, 2005). The effect may be closely related to the intervention under study, for example, falls averted when evaluating fall prevention (Farag et al, 2016) or can also be more general, for example, life-years saved (Jutkowitz et al, 2012). A variant of cost-effectiveness analysis is cost-utility analysis. The specific feature of a cost-utility analysis is the use of quality-adjusted life-years (QALYs), including a combination of the time perspective and health-related quality of life (HRQoL) (Drummond et al, 2005). Some commonly used instruments to measure HRQoL are EQ-5D and SF-12. In the calculation of QALYs, data on HRQoL and a time interval are combined (for example, 1 year in full health is equal to one QALY). The actual difference between cost-utility and cost-effectiveness can easily be seen in Figure 7.1. Considering life-years gained as the unit of effect, the difference between interventions A and B is the difference on the *x*-axis (cost-effectiveness), whereas the difference in QALYs includes the whole area between the curves (cost-utility).

The concepts of cost-utility and cost-effectiveness are often confused in the literature. For simplicity, we will use the concept of cost-effectiveness analysis throughout this chapter and clearly state when QALYs is the outcome used.

One way of presenting results from a cost-effectiveness analysis is by using the cost-effectiveness plane in which differences in costs and health outcomes

Figure 7.1: Development of HRQoL over time in relation to two different interventions

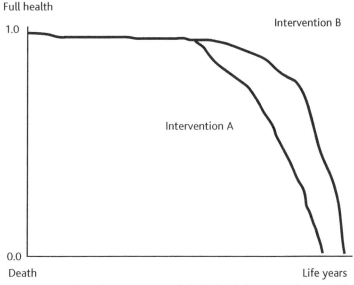

Note: Intervention B results in the maintenance of a higher level of HRQoL and postponed mortality compared to intervention A (which also could be no intervention). The QALYs gained are represented by the area between the curves.

Source: Zingmark (2015)

between alternative treatments are plotted in a graph; health outcomes are usually plotted on the *x*-axis and costs on the *y*-axis. The graphic presentation has four quadrants, as shown later in Figure 7.2. The northwest quadrant represents greater costs and smaller effects, while the southeast quadrant represents greater effects and smaller costs. If, for example, the reablement intervention results in larger health gains and higher costs compared to usual care, the study should be placed in the northeast quadrant.

Cost-benefit analysis

Cost-benefit analysis widens the concept of value by expressing the intervention consequences in monetary terms which help facilitate a comparison of program costs (Drummond et al, 2005). This means that the outcome effects described previously for cost-effectiveness analysis such as falls averted, life-years saved, or for cost-utility analysis, QALYs gained, need to be translated into monetary values to allow interpretation alongside the costs. The cost-benefit analysis also makes it possible to identify whether one intervention offers an overall net welfare gain, and how the net welfare gain for that intervention compares to alternate interventions (Palmer et al, 1999). Using interventions with the greatest net gain will increase efficiency.

Time perspectives in health economic evaluation

The time horizon chosen for the analysis is an important feature of any evaluation, meaning that we are most often interested in looking at the effect of reablement after 3 months or a longer period, say 12 months, which may indicate whether effects can be considered sustainable. For the purpose of health economic evaluation, the time horizon needs to be chosen so that all relevant health effects and costs that the intervention may impact are captured. As stated, the benefit of using QALYs as an outcome is that the accumulated effects on HRQoL in combination with time is captured. The time horizon is also central in the calculation of costs. The data for estimating QALYs and costs can be part of ordinary data collection and therefore limited to the time horizon of a clinical trial (Drummond et al, 2005). Potential long-term gains on HRQoL or costs will in such cases not be included, which could be considered problematic. For example, there is a risk that the full costs for implementing an intervention are included; whereas, the long-term effects and costs are not included. In a study by Flood et al (2005) comparing assessment and subsequent actions made by occupational therapists and social workers, the costs for home adaptations were included, but not the long-term effects for quality of life and costs related to dependency. Especially for an intervention such as reablement, aiming to increase a person's health and to maintain their ability to engage in daily activities, the effects obtained during the trial period may extend beyond the period of the actual trial. Thus, the time horizon for health economic evaluations in reablement is an important feature that needs to be considered in relation to the trial design.

Trial designs

In relation to health economic evaluation, two different trial designs are common: a randomised controlled trial (RCT) design and a model-based design. RCTs are often conducted to evaluate the effects of an intervention in relation to a comparator (such as a different intervention) and for the purpose of health economic evaluation, specific data on health outcomes and costs can be added (Drummond et al, 2005). Two features that are important to consider in relation to RCTs and health economic evaluation are the time horizon, as mentioned previously, and the statistical power to detect differences. If the RCT was designed for the purpose of evaluating effects on a specific health outcome, the sample size, that is number of participants, may not be sufficiently large to detect differences in costs. Thus, these aspects need to be considered at the planning stages of an RCT that includes a health economic evaluation.

An alternative design to an RCT is decision analytic modelling, in which information from different sources is combined into models, for example, decision trees or Markov models (Drummond et al, 2005; Briggs et al, 2006). The model represents a realistic scenario for different health events to occur, including probabilities that these events will occur in the presence of no intervention or if an intervention is implemented (Briggs et al, 2006). Thus, the impact on health and costs over time if no intervention is implemented can be compared to the impact if it is implemented. Furthermore, the time horizon can be extended over a sufficiently long time period to capture relevant health effects and use of resources when a model approach is used.

A summary of existing evidence of the cost-effectiveness of reablement

Following the introduction to health economic evaluation methods, we explore in the following sections the evidence of the cost-effectiveness of reablement.

Methods

Based on the aim to summarise what is known from the existing literature about the cost-effectiveness of reablement in relation to traditional home care, the existing evidence was explored. Although a formal scoping review was not conducted, the process was guided by the framework for scoping reviews proposed by Arksey and O'Malley (2005).

Identification of focus points for the health economic evaluation of reablement

For the decision on how to assess and compare the health outcomes and costs of different reablement studies, we were guided by the CHEERS framework. Since 2013, the CHEERS statement provides a reporting standard for health economic evaluations (Husereau et al, 2013), similar to the CONSORT statement for RCTs (Moher et al, 2010). For the purpose of this chapter, eight items from the CHEERS statement were selected to guide the health-economic comparison of reablement studies:

1. For which target population have interventions been evaluated?
2. In which settings and locations have health economic perspectives of reablement been evaluated?
3. From which study perspective have health economic evaluations been conducted?
4. In relation to which comparators have interventions been evaluated?
5. Which time horizons have been applied in the existing literature?
6. In relation to which health outcomes have health economic evaluations been conducted?
7. Which costs have been included in existing health economic studies?
8. Have interventions been cost-effective?

Adjustments to the same currency and price date

In addition, the calculation and comparison of intervention costs were based on the year of original publication and were adjusted for inflation until 2020 and converted to Euros (€) (for the purpose of this chapter based on the currency in December 2018).

Identifying and selecting relevant studies

In collaboration with a University librarian, a brief literature search was conducted in September 2018 and an updated literature search was conducted in May 2020, including databases such as Medline, Embase, Cinahl, and Web of Science. Search words included reablement, restorative care, function-focused care, active service model, and enablement, combined with terms like cost-effectiveness, cost-effect, economic evaluation, cost-utility analysis, and cost-benefit analysis. Titles and abstracts from 70 potential references were screened and selected full texts were read as a whole. In addition, the Reable international network members were contacted via email for additional references. Studies included were based on a consensus discussion involving all three authors.

Economic studies of reablement/restorative care with a control group published with or without peer-reviewing in English or a Scandinavian language reporting results were included. Studies of other rehabilitation interventions and early discharge as intervention were excluded.

Charting data and reporting results

Based on the research question, in line with the selected CHEERS items, all results were charted in a table, see Table 7.1.

Findings

Eight studies were included (Table7.1). Five studies were peer-reviewed publications including two RCTs, two model-based studies, and one retrospective cohort study (Lewin et al, 2013; Lewin et al, 2014; Kjerstad and Tuntland, 2016; Zingmark et al, 2017; Bauer et al, 2019). Three studies were grey literature reports (McLeod and Mair, 2009; Glendinning et al, 2010; Langeland et al, 2016).

Target group

The total number of participants was 13,191 spanning from 45 to 10,368 participants found in six of the eight studies. The studies by Zingmark et al (2017) and Bauer et al (2019) were model-based in which estimates of cost-effectiveness were based on published data from a range of studies. The mean age across the studies was 79.9 ($\pm$8.4) years, with participant ages ranging from 19 through to 101 years. None of the studies conducted sub-group analyses and could therefore not conclude whether reablement is more cost-effective according to age, gender and so on.

Setting and location

Two studies were undertaken in Norway (Kjerstad and Tuntland, 2016; Langeland et al, 2016), two in Australia (Lewin et al, 2013; Lewin et al, 2014), one in Scotland (McLeod and Mair, 2009), two in England (Glendinning et al, 2010; Bauer et al, 2019) and the Swedish modelling study (Zingmark et al, 2017) utilised data on the intervention effect on independence in personal activities of daily living from Australia. All studies were conducted in primary or community care/municipality settings, including rural and urban municipalities/regions.

Table 7.1: Identified health economic papers including grey and peer-reviewed literature

Study (authors, year, and publication type)	Country, setting, study design, perspective of analysis	Population	Intervention	Comparator	Health outcomes	Included costs	Cost-effectiveness and time horizon
Bauer et al (2019) Peer-reviewed publication.	Based on data from England. Markov model including three states ('alive at home with care'; 'alive at home without care'; and 'care home admission or death'). National Health Services (NHS) and Personal Social Services (PSS) perspective.	Two hypothetical cohorts of 1000 people each: one cohort received reablement and the other cohort received standard home care.	An inter-disciplinary team carried out comprehensive multidimensional assessment and goal-oriented care planning in partnership with the person who used the service and their family and carers. The intervention effect was based on Lewin (2013a, 2014) because it was deemed sufficiently similar to the UK.	Traditional home care services.	No health outcome included.	Home care use (home care and reablement costs). Overhead costs (for example management, buildings) were included. Healthcare usage (hospital admission costs).	Cost-minimisation analysis. Costs were included from a life-time perspective and the intervention implemented at different ages. The intervention cost was estimated at €3,275 (lower bound: €2,375; upper bound: €4,715). 3.5 per cent discount in the first year was applied. Mean costs per person were €68,297 in the reablement group and €70,788 in the control group. The mean difference was –€2,491 in favour of reablement. Overall probability that reablement was cost-reducing was 94.5%. The potential cost savings in all scenarios was >€1,209 per person.

Table 7.1: Identified health economic papers including grey and peer-reviewed literature (continued)

Study (authors, year, and publication type)	Country, setting, study design, perspective of analysis	Population	Intervention	Comparator	Health outcomes	Included costs	Cost-effectiveness and time horizon
Glendinning et al (2010) Grey literature.	England, ten unspecified study sites, five for each arm of the study. Prospective clinical controlled trial. Societal perspective.	In total 1,015 participants, 654 in the reablement group, and 361 in the control group. Mean age 80 years, age span 29–101 years. Participants referred from community/ hospital to reablement or traditional home care services.	Team-based reablement (variation between sites which professionals were included). Focus on supporting participants to develop confidence and relearn self-care skills, may include equipment. Duration, normally up to 6 weeks.	Traditional home care services.	Health-related quality of life (EQ-5D) and social care- related quality of life (ASCOT)	Salaries related to social care and healthcare. Unit costs for healthcare services. Overhead costs (for example management, offices). Informal care costs were not included.	Cost-effectiveness was established over 12 months. The cost for a reablement episode was €2,198. Reablement was associated with a significant decrease in social care service use; 60% less than the comparator group. The social care cost (including reablement) was €3,393 compared to €3,923 for social care only, the difference was not significant. Also, when healthcare costs were included, there was no significant difference in total costs. Reablement was cost-effective in relation to EQ-5D scores, particularly when only including social care, still effective when including healthcare costs also. The results were more modest in relation to ASCOT scores. At a willingness to pay threshold of €22,500/ QALY, the probability of reablement being cost-effective was 98%.

(continued)

145

Table 7.1: Identified health economic papers including grey and peer-reviewed literature (continued)

Study (authors, year, and publication type)	Country, setting, study design, perspective of analysis	Population	Intervention	Comparator	Health outcomes	Included costs	Cost-effectiveness and time horizon
Kjerstad and Tuntland (2016) Peer-reviewed publication.	Norway. Rural municipality in Western Norway. A prospective randomised controlled trial. Municipality perspective.	In total, 45 participants, 25 in intervention group, 21 in control group. Mean age 79.9 and 78.1 years respectively.	Focus on improving independent functioning in daily activities identified as important by the participant, time-limited (that is average 10 weeks), person-centred, delivered by multidisciplinary team in the home or community.	Traditional home care services.	Self-perceived activity performance and satisfaction with performance evaluated with the Canadian Occupational Performance Measure (COPM) on a scale from 1–10 (best).	Daily registration of usage of home-based personnel. Mean (SD) costs per visit, mean number of visits, mean cost per participant. Total costs, average costs.	Cost-effectiveness was established over 9 months. Average cost difference per participant approx. €123 lower for reablement during the intervention period. Both COPM performance and satisfaction scores were significantly improved at 3 months in favour of reablement. From 3–9 months, the intervention group requested significantly fewer home visits and of shorter duration compared with control group. The mean costs per participant were €704 and €1,515 for reablement and control group respectively; the difference being €813. ICER (cost per COPM point gained) was lower for the reablement group compared to the control by €95 (performance) and €72 (satisfaction). In conclusion, reablement was found to be more cost-effective than usual care.

Table 7.1: Identified health economic papers including grey and peer-reviewed literature (continued)

Study (authors, year, and publication type)	Country, setting, study design, perspective of analysis	Population	Intervention	Comparator	Health outcomes	Included costs	Cost-effectiveness and time horizon
Langeland et al (2016) Grey literature.	Norway, primary care settings involving 43 municipalities from South to North of Norway. Multi-center, prospective clinical controlled trial. Societal perspective.	In total 833 participants, 712 in reablement group, 129 in control group. Mean age 78 years, age span 19–97 years.	Focus on improving independent functioning in daily activities identified as important by the participant, time-limited on average 5 weeks, person-centred, delivered by multidisciplinary team in the home or community.	Traditional home care services.	Health-related quality of Life (EQ-5D-5L) and quality adjusted life years (QALY).	Costs were divided into three groups: 1. resources related to reablement (weekly registrations of work hours); 2. resources related to healthcare services in primary care not included in reablement (GP visits, practical care, nurses, physiotherapy, occupational therapy); 3. resources related to hospitalisations, rehabilitation in institutions and use of specialist and outpatient care.	Cost-effectiveness was established over 6 months. HRQoL was significantly improved at 6 months in favour of reablement. In terms of QALYs gained, the effect was 0.015 (p-value = 0.04). In cost group 1 costs were higher in the reablement group from baseline and the following 5–6 weeks. In the following months until week 23 costs were lower for reablement. From week 24 and onwards the costs were similar in both groups. Cost group 2 and 3 did not differ between groups. In all, the difference in costs was €106 per participant. Based on cost group 1 ICER (cost per QALY gained) was €7,007.

(continued)

Table 7.1: Identified health economic papers including grey and peer-reviewed literature (continued)

Study (authors, year, and publication type)	Country, setting, study design, perspective of analysis	Population	Intervention	Comparator	Health outcomes	Included costs	Cost-effectiveness and time horizon
Lewin et al (2013) Peer-reviewed publication	Australia, in regional and metropolitan areas of Western Australia. Services provided by Silver Chain, a private not-for-profit home care provider. Retrospective cohort study. Municipality perspective.	In total 10,368 older adults, 8,036 in two reablement groups, 2,332 in control group. Home Independence Program (HIP, $n = 2586$) referred from the community. Personal Enablement Program (PEP, $n = 5450$) referred from hospital. Mean age total sample 78.1 years.	Short-term, individualised, goal-oriented, focused on promoting independence and active engagement in daily living activities through task analysis, assistive technology and design. HIP 12-week limit, PEP 8-week limit.	Traditional home care services (HACC).	No health outcome included.	Home care costs. Data sourced from Western Australia Department of Health, using 2009 unit costs as the metric.	A cost-analysis was conducted over 57 months (4 years and 9 months). Median cost of home care in reablement groups (57 months): PEP: €3,123; HIP: €3,268. Cost of home care in comparator group (HACC) (57 months): €11,801. Median saving per person of PEP and HIP was €8,679 and €8,533 respectively.

Table 7.1: Identified health economic papers including grey and peer-reviewed literature (continued)

Study (authors, year, and publication type)	Country, setting, study design, perspective of analysis	Population	Intervention	Comparator	Health outcomes	Included costs	Cost-effectiveness and time horizon
Lewin et al (2014) Peer-reviewed publication.	Australia, in the Perth metropolitan area in the state of Western Australia. Services provided by Silver Chain. Retrospective randomised controlled trial. Societal perspective.	In total 750 older adults, 375 in each group. Mean age HACC 82.7 years; HIP 81.8 years (for ITT analysis).	Home Independence Program (HIP) is a short-term, individualised, goal oriented program, which promotes independence and active engagement in daily living activities through task analysis, assistive technology, and design. 12-week limit.	Traditional home care services (HACC).	No health outcome included.	Aged care use (HACC services and HACC costs). Healthcare usage (emergency department presentations and unplanned inpatient admissions and costs). Total costs are the sum of costs in each setting.	A costs analysis was conducted over 2 years. The mean total cost was significantly lower by a factor of 0.83 for the reablement group: Reablement: €12,702; Comparator: €15,588. Reablement clients vs comparator: - used fewer home care hours (mean [SD] 117.3 [129.4] vs 191.2 [230.4]); - were less likely to be approved for a higher level of aged care (n [%], 171 [55.2] vs 249 [63.0]); - less likely to go to emergency department (OR = 0.69, 95% CI = 0.50–0.94); - were less likely to have an unplanned hospital admission (OR 0.69, 95% CI = 0.50–0.95).

(continued)

149

Table 7.1: Identified health economic papers including grey and peer-reviewed literature (continued)

Study (authors, year, and publication type)	Country, setting, study design, perspective of analysis	Population	Intervention	Comparator	Health outcomes	Included costs	Cost-effectiveness and time horizon
McLeod and Mair (2009) Grey literature	Edinburgh municipality, Scotland. Prospective clinical controlled trial. Municipality perspective.	In total 180 older adults, 90 per group. Mean age not reported. Participants referred from community/hospital to reablement matched with a group receiving traditional home care services.	Team-based reablement including service manager, care coordinator, OT, home care organiser, administration staff and social care workers. Focus on participants' strengths and abilities, and including them as an active participant in the process. Duration 6 weeks but occasionally more extensive.	Traditional home care services.	No health outcome included.	Weekly care costs (social care worker/home help/ independent sector), management/ supervisory, and administration costs, weekly OT costs, training costs (where applicable).	A cost-analysis was conducted over 6 weeks. Reablement reduced the total hours of care by 41% over the 6 weeks whereas the comparison group required a small increase in hours of care over the 6 weeks. Intervention costs was estimated to €130. The mean total cost was lower in the comparison group: Reablement: €1,534 per client; Comparator: €1,183 per client.

Table 7.1: Identified health economic papers including grey and peer-reviewed literature (continued)

Study (authors, year, and publication type)	Country, setting, study design, perspective of analysis	Population	Intervention	Comparator	Health outcomes	Included costs	Cost-effectiveness and time horizon
Zingmark et al (2017) Peer-reviewed publication	Based on data from Canada, Sweden, Hong Kong (China), and Western Australia (Australia). Municipality settings. Markov model including 4 states of dependency (mild, moderate, severe, total and, death). Societal perspective.	Hypothetical cohort of community-dwelling older adults with a bathing disability.	Focus on improving a person's ability to perform self-care tasks related to bathing. Also includes technical aids when necessary. The intervention effect was based on Lewin et al, 2014 and implemented as a 40% increased probability of regaining independence in self-care in the first year.	Traditional home care services.	QALYs and HRQoL scores (for each state based on previously published literature (including EQ-5D and Health Utility Index.)	Societal costs for each state including: formal health and social care (home help, special accommodation) and informal care. Intervention cost: salaries, technical equipment.	Cost-effectiveness was established over 8 years. Intervention costs were estimated to €128. After 8 years the intervention resulted in 0.052 QALYS gained and reduced societal costs by €2,410 per person. A sensitivity analysis indicated that the intervention effect had a large impact on cost-effectiveness whereas intervention cost only had a small impact on cost effectiveness. Conclusion: the intervention targeting bathing disability among older adults is a cost-effective use of resources and leads to QALY gains and reduced societal costs over 8 years.

Study perspectives and estimated costs

Three studies considered costs from a municipality perspective including a comparison of costs related to home care and the intervention (McLeod and Mair, 2009; Lewin et al, 2013; Kjerstad and Tuntland, 2016). One study was conducted from a service provider perspective (Bauer et al, 2019). Four studies included costs from a societal perspective (Glendinning et al, 2010; Lewin et al, 2014; Langeland et al, 2016; Zingmark et al, 2017). In three of these, healthcare costs were included in addition to more direct home care and intervention costs. In addition to health and social care costs, one study also included costs related to the value of the time for informal care (Zingmark et al, 2017).

Comparators

All studies evaluated a reablement service in relation to conventional home care. However, the models of service delivery and skills mix did vary. In addition, and as we outline in the following, there were some variations in how the reablement interventions were studied, such as the time horizon, the choice of health outcomes, and the choice of cost-effectiveness method applied.

Time horizon

The time horizon varied greatly between the studies. A short time horizon of 6 weeks was applied in one study (McLeod and Mair, 2009), a medium to long time horizon was applied in three studies, of 6 months (Kjerstad and Tuntland, 2016) and 12 months (Glendinning et al, 2010; Langeland et al, 2016). In four studies, the time horizon was more extended, for example 2 years (Lewin et al, 2014), 57 months (Lewin et al, 2013), 8 years (Zingmark et al, 2017), and a lifetime perspective (Bauer et al, 2019).

Choice of health outcomes

Four studies did not include any health outcomes at all (McLeod and Mair, 2009; Lewin et al, 2013; Lewin et al, 2014; Bauer et al, 2019), whereas the other four studies included various health outcomes. Three studies included health-related quality of life (EQ-5D) (Glendinning et al, 2010; Langeland et al, 2016; Zingmark et al, 2017) and one study included social care-related quality of life (ASCOT) (Glendinning et al, 2010). Two studies included quality-adjusted life-years (QALYs) (Langeland et al, 2016; Zingmark et al, 2017) and one study included occupational performance and satisfaction with that performance (COPM) (Kjerstad and Tuntland, 2016).

Cost-effectiveness

Four studies focused on the comparison of costs (McLeod and Mair, 2009; Lewin et al, 2013; Lewin et al, 2014; Bauer et al, 2019), whereas four included full health economic evaluations (Glendinning et al, 2010; Kjerstad and Tuntland, 2016; Langeland et al, 2016; Zingmark et al, 2017). Four studies found reablement to be a cost-effective intervention in a time perspective from 6 months to 8 years (Glendinning et al, 2010; Kjerstad and Tuntland, 2016; Langeland et al, 2016; Zingmark et al, 2017). For example, in the study by Kjerstad and Tuntland (2016), the intervention resulted in positive effects on ADL and significantly fewer home visits over a period of 3 months, resulting in slightly lower costs compared to usual care. In addition, four studies found that reablement resulted in a reduction of health and/or social care costs in a perspective from 2 years or more (Lewin et al, 2013; Lewin et al, 2014; Zingmark et al, 2017; Bauer et al, 2019). For example, in the retrospective study by Lewin et al (2013) including data on more than 10,000 clients, the results clearly showed how the differences in median costs for home care between reablement and usual care continued to diverge over a period of 57 months indicating that reablement resulted in 28 per cent of the cost for usual care at the end of the period. In contrast, one study found that reablement was more costly than conventional traditional home care services over a 6-week period (McLeod and Mair, 2009). Figure 7.2 provides a cost-effectiveness plane where the included studies are inserted. As can be

Figure 7.2: The cost-effectiveness plane for the included studies

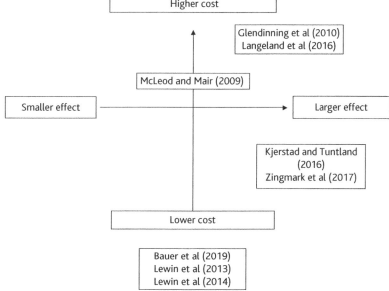

seen in Figure 7.2 it is the two studies of Kjerstad and Tuntland (2016) and Zingmark et al (2017) that show the highest degree of cost-effectiveness.

General discussion

As for related fields (Lambert et al, 2014), we found that the numbers of health economic studies of reablement were few. Our findings indicate that health economic perspectives on reablement are limited to studies conducted in the UK and Scandinavia. If cost-analysis is also considered, another two trials from Australia are added to the evidence base.

In all studies included here, reablement was evaluated in relation to usual care, that is conventional home care, and in all studies except one, reablement resulted in positive effects on outcomes covering quality of life and performance of daily activities and/or lower costs. It should be noted, however, that the variety of health outcomes evaluated, and the costs included, make comparisons between studies difficult. Also, in Chapter 5 by Lewin et al and in Chapter 6 by Tuntland et al the authors discuss the wide variety of client level outcomes used in previous reablement research. Regarding costs, only one study included costs related to both healthcare, social care, and informal care whereas three trials were limited to only municipality costs. Whereas different study perspectives can be justified, the actual choice of perspective will affect which specific costs are included. Subsequently, the results need to be interpreted accordingly and the possibility of comparing cost-effectiveness between trials is limited. In general, however, a societal perspective is recommended, and as such, all relevant costs should be included. Since reablement potentially can affect the need a person has for health and social care services as well as informal care, it is reasonable to recommend applying a societal perspective for future health economic evaluations. If all relevant societal costs were to be included in health economic evaluations of reablement, the results would provide a broader and more reliable picture of how reablement impacts resource use and costs. In addition, for the purpose of decision-making, a societal perspective would provide a broader base of information when reablement is prioritised in relation to other alternatives on how to use existing resources.

Noteworthy is the similarity in intervention costs, approximately €130, in the studies by Mcleod and Mair (2009) and Zingmark et al (2017). In contrast, Glendinning et al (2010) and Bauer et al (2019) reported the costs for a reablement period to be in the span of €2,198–3,100. The large difference in the estimated cost for the intervention is explained by which costs were included. It goes beyond the purpose of this chapter to discuss issues related to costing in detail, but how costs are identified, measured, and valued is a central feature of health economic evaluation that needs to be clearly reported (Husereau et al, 2013). As shown by Glendinning et al (2010), the costs for salaries constitute the largest costs for reablement (64 per cent), but also overhead costs (for example management, supervision, offices, buildings), when considered, constitute a significant proportion of the overall costs. In addition to the costs included, the time perspective is central to the understanding of costs and subsequently plays a role as the nominator in the cost-effectiveness equation. It should be noted, however, that costs related to the intervention mainly occur during the first weeks or months from baseline and are low in relation to other costs such as home care, especially since such costs accumulate over time (Lewin et al, 2013; Lindholm et al, 2013).

Three studies only included economic outcomes. While a costs analysis can be relevant, it should be noted, that such studies are not considered full health economic evaluations (Drummond et al, 2005). When considering how best to use available resources, the recommendation is that health outcomes also need to be included. However, as argued in the study by Bauer et al (2019) there is a lack of evidence as to whether reablement results in any health effects compared to care as usual, and thus a cost-minimisation analysis, only including a comparison of costs, is highly relevant for decision-makers.

In contrast to the five studies that applied a prospective design, three studies were retrospective and used data previously collected or published (Lewin et al, 2013; Zingmark et al, 2017; Bauer et al, 2019). Given the complexity of conducting prospective studies and the time before results can be presented, retrospective study designs can also provide valuable information. The time horizons used in the studies using a retrospective design, for example, 6–8 years, would likely be challenging in a prospective study. The study by Zingmark et al (2017), provided the first model-based reablement study extrapolating the impact on health effects and societal costs by applying a time horizon of 8 years. Lewin et al (2013) used register data showing cost differences between reablement and usual home care over 57 months. Retrospective and model-based studies are not common within the field of reablement, but from a broader perspective, model-based studies are the most commonly used method in cost–utility analysis (Wisløff et al, 2014). Although not a health economic study, a study by Cook et al provided another example of a modelling study. They included almost 100,000 clients receiving occupational therapy and physiotherapy in a home care context. The results showed the benefits of interventions in terms of positive transitions between different health states displayed in a Markov model, that is increased chances for recovery and reduced risk for negative transitions over 63 months (2013). Taken together, there are different possible approaches to extend the time horizon over a longer period than would be feasible in a prospective randomised controlled trial.

Recommendations for clinicians and decision-makers

The health and cost outcomes used varied between the included studies. This makes a comparison of results difficult and conclusions vague. The models of service delivery and skills-mix of the reablement intervention also varied between the included studies. No studies evaluated the effects of different models of service delivery but compared reablement with the national/local model of home care. Hence, it is unclear whether the interventions are comparable across countries. As a consequence, the external validity of the findings may be uncertain. The actual content of the reablement intervention is likely to vary between studies, even though the overall purpose is similar. The number of home visits and sessions for supervision of home care staff are features of the reablement intervention that will have an impact on the costs of the intervention. Precisely how the reablement intervention is delivered is also likely to impact on the quality of the intervention. Thus, the question of whether a more extensive intervention produces better outcomes is relevant and should be explored in future studies. However, Zingmark et al showed that the actual costs for the intervention had a very small impact on overall cost-effectiveness; instead, the most critical feature was the intervention effect, that is, whether the person gained improvements in independent performance in daily activities or any of the other outcome goals included (Zingmark et al, 2017). Thus, if a more extensive intervention, for example, additional home visits, could further improve health outcomes, then the additional intervention costs would likely be justified.

In all, six out of eight studies indicated that reablement was cost-effective or resulted in lower costs in relation to traditional home care services. The time frame (6 weeks) in the study by McLeod and Mair (2009) might have been too short to detect any cost savings. We acknowledge that this chapter is not a systematic review, nor has a meta-analysis or risk of bias assessment of included studies been conducted. In addition, the number of health economic studies in the field of reablement is very low. Hence, the following recommendation must be interpreted with caution. However, based on the results in this chapter, reablement appears to be a cost-effective intervention. Supported in addition by two systematic reviews (Faria, 2016; Flemming et al, 2021), decision-makers and clinicians might consider implementing reablement in their respective regions or municipalities.

Recommendations for researchers

Three of the included studies were not published in peer-reviewed scientific journals, of which two of the controlled trials used non-randomised data and were at risk of selection bias (Glendinning et al, 2010; Langeland et al, 2016). Hence, the evidence in these studies is considered to be of insufficient quality. With only two randomised controlled trials published (Lewin et al, 2014; Kjerstad and Tuntland, 2016), there is a marked lack of high-quality RCTs conducting health economic evaluations on reablement. In line with research on health promotion and prevention for older people (Bajraktari et al, 2020), there are also few health economic evaluation studies in the field of reablement. Thus, the basis for decision-makers is limited and more research is urgently needed. While health economic evaluation methods require additional data to be collected, such data can relatively easily be added to study protocols at the planning stage of effectiveness studies. Thereby, important research questions related to cost-effectiveness of reablement could be addressed and the basis for decision-making would be improved. Future research should consider using a more rigorous study design with a larger study sample and publish the results in peer-reviewed journals. Also, retrospective designs should be considered in which already existing data can be used. Independent of study design, the CHEERS statement provides valuable guidance on a range of aspects that should be considered in the planning and reporting of studies.

Finally, incremental cost-effectiveness ratios (ICER) as recommended by the CHEERS checklist (Husereau et al, 2013), were only reported in two studies (Kjerstad and Tuntland, 2016; Langeland et al, 2016). Moreover, no subgroup analyses, for instance in terms of diagnoses or level of functional limitations in participants, were conducted in any of the eight studies. As further investigated in Chapter 8 by Rahja and Thuesen, reablement is often aimed at persons with only limited functional limitations rather than persons with dementia/cognitive impairment. Future health economic evaluations should consider conducting subgroup analyses to identify groups of individuals for whom the intervention is more or less favourable, to prevent the intervention from being offered to populations in which it is not cost-effective (Faria, 2016). For such analyses to be possible, sample sizes need to be sufficiently large. Thus, in order to expand the evidence on health economic perspectives in reablement, researchers need to conduct trials with larger samples and rigorously choose outcomes from a societal perspective including costs related to health-, social- and informal care.

Conclusion

Reablement has been viewed as an answer to several enduring challenges in health and social care, including a means to promote health and independence among older people as well as to reduce the societal costs related to fast-growing older populations. This chapter has described health economic evaluation methods and trial designs used in health economic evaluations. Based on a literature review and a summary of the existing evidence, reablement is found to be a promising cost-effective intervention compared to usual home care services. However, the number of publications including health economic perspectives on reablement is very low and results must be interpreted with caution. Additional studies are urgently needed to improve knowledge on health economic perspectives on reablement and to improve the basis for decision-makers.

Acknowledgements

We thank University Librarian Gunhild Austrheim for conducting the literature searches.

References

Arksey, H. and O'Malley, L. (2005) 'Scoping studies: towards a methodological framework', *International Journal of Social Research Methodology*, 8(1): 19–32.

Aspinal, F., Glasby, J., Rostgaard, T., Tuntland, H., and Westendorp, R. (2016) 'Reablement: supporting older people towards independence', *Age and Ageing*, 45(5): 574–8.

Bajraktari, S., Sandlund, M., and Zingmark, M. (2020) 'Health-promoting and preventive interventions for community-dwelling older people published from inception to 2019: a scoping review to guide decision making in a Swedish municipality context', *Archives of Public Health*, 78: 97.

Bauer, A., Fernandez, J.L., Henderson, C., Wittenberg, R., and Knapp, M. (2019) 'Cost-minimisation analysis of home care reablement for older people in England: A modelling study', *Health & Social Care in the Community*, 27(5): 1241–50.

Briggs, A.H., Claxton, K., and Sculpher, M.J. (2006) *Decision Modelling for Health Economic Evaluation*, Oxford: Oxford University Press.

Cook, R.J., Berg, K., Lee, K.-A., Poss, J.W., Hirdes, J.P. and Stolee, P. (2013) 'Rehabilitation in home care is associated with functional improvement and preferred discharge', *Archives of Physical Medicine and Rehabilitation*, 94(6): 1038–47.

Drummond, M.F., Schulpher, M.J., Torrance, G.W., O'Brien, B.J., and Stoddart, G.L. (2005) *Methods for the Economic Evaluation of Health Care Programmes*, 3rd edn, Oxford: Oxford University Press.

Farag, I., Sherrington, C., Hayes, A., Canning, C.G., Lord, S.R., Close, J.C., Fung, V.S., and Howard, K. (2016) 'Economic evaluation of a falls prevention exercise program among people with Parkinson's disease', *Movement Disorders*, 31(1): 53–61.

Faria, R. (2016) 'Economic evaluation of social care interventions: lessons drawn from a systematic review of the methods used to evaluate reablement', *Health Economics & Outcome Research: Open Access*, 2: 107.

Flemming, J., Armijo-Olivo, S., Dennett, L., Lapointe, P., Robertson, D., Wang, J. et al (2021) 'Enhanced home care interventions for community residing adults compared with usual care on health and cost-effectiveness outcomes: a systematic review', *American Journal of Physical Medicine & Rehabilitation*, 100(9): 906–17.

Flood, C., Mugford, M., Stewart, S., Harvey, I., Poland, F., and Lloyd-Smith, W. (2005) 'Occupational therapy compared with social work assessment for older people. An economic evaluation alongside the CAMELOT randomised controlled trial', *Age & Ageing*, 34(1): 47–52.

Glendinning, C., Jones, K., Baxter, K., Rabiee, P., Curtis, L.A., Wilde, A., Arksey, H., and Forder, J.E. (2010) *Home Care Re-ablement Services: Investigating the Longer-term Impacts (Prospective Longitudinal Study)*, York/Canterburry: Social Policy Research Unit (SPRU)/Personal Social Service Research Unit (PSSRU).

Husereau, D., Drummond, M., Petrou, S., Carswell, C., Moher, D., Greenberg, D., Augustovski, F., Briggs, A.H., Mauskopf, J., Loder, E., and Force, C.T. (2013) 'Consolidated Health Economic Evaluation Reporting Standards (CHEERS) statement', *British Medical Journal*, 346: f1049.

Jutkowitz, E., Gitlin, L.N., Pizzi, L.T., Lee, E., and Dennis, M.P. (2012) 'Cost effectiveness of a home-based intervention that helps functionally vulnerable older adults age in place at home', *Journal of Aging Research*, 2012: 680265.

Kjerstad, E. and Tuntland, H. (2016) 'Reablement in community-dwelling older adults: a cost-effectiveness study analysis alongside a randomized controlled trial', *Health Economics Review*, 6(15): 1–10.

Lambert, R., Radford, K., Smyth, G., Morley, M., and Ahmed-Landeryou, M. (2014) 'Occupational therapy can flourish in the 21st century – a case for professional engagement with health economics', *The British Journal of Occupational Therapy*, 77(5): 260–3.

Langeland, E., Førland, O., Aas, E., Birkeland, A., Folkestad, B., Kjeken, I., Jacobsen, F., and Tuntland, H. (2016) 'Modeller for hverdagsrehabilitering – en følgeevaluering i norske kommuner. Effekter for brukerne og gevinster for kommunene?' ['Models of reablement. A study in Norwegian muncipalities. Effects for users and gains for municipalities?'], Report, Senter for omsorgsforskning vest, Høgskolen i Bergen, CHARM.

Lewin, G., Alfonso, H., and Alan, J. (2013) 'Evidence for the long term cost effectiveness of home care reablement programs', *Clinical Intervention in Aging*, 8: 1273–81.

Lewin, G., Allan, J., Patterson, C., Knuima, M., Boldy, D., and Hendrie, D. (2014) 'A comparison of the home-care and healthcare service use and costs of older Australians randomised to receive a restorative or a conventional home-care service', *Health & Social Care in the Community*, 22(3): 328–36.

Lindholm, C., Gustavsson, A., Jönsson, L., and Wimo, A. (2013) 'Costs explained by function rather than diagnosis – results from the SNAC Nordanstig elderly cohort in Sweden', *International Journal of Geriatric Psychiatry*, 28(5): 454–62.

McLeod, B. and Mair, M. (2009) *Evaluation of City of Edinburgh Council Home Care Re-Ablement Service*, Edinburgh: Scottish Government Social Research.

Moher, D., Hopewell, S., Schulz, K.F., Montori, V., Gøtzsche, P.C., Devereaux, P.J., Elbourne, D., Egger, M., Altman, D.G., and Consolidated Standards of Reporting Trials Group (2010) 'CONSORT 2010 explanation and elaboration: updated guidelines for reporting parallel group randomised trials', *Journal of Clinical Epidemiology*, 63(8): e1–37.

Palmer, S., Byford, S., and Raftery, J. (1999) 'Economics notes: types of economic evaluation', *BMJ: British Medical Journal*, 318(7194): 1349.

Wisløff, T., Hagen, G., Hamidi, V., Movik, E., Klemp, M., and Olsen, J.A. (2014) 'Estimating QALY gains in applied studies: a review of cost-utility analyses published in 2010', *Pharmacoeconomics*, 32(4): 367–75.

Zingmark, M. (2015) 'Occupation-focused and occupation-based interventions for community-dwelling older people: intervention effects in relation to facets of occupational engagement and cost effectiveness', Sweden: Department of Community Medicine and Rehabilitation, Occupational Therapy Medical Dissertations, Umeå University.

Zingmark, M., Nilsson, I., Norström, F., Sahlén, K.G., and Lindholm, L. (2017) 'Cost effectiveness of an intervention focused on reducing bathing disability', *European Journal of Ageing*, 14(3): 233–41.

PART III

Experience

8

Reablement and dementia

Miia Rahja and Jette Thuesen

Introduction

Dementia is the leading cause of dependency and disability among older individuals (World Health Organization, 2012). While the reablement approach is increasingly being integrated in aged care, this has not been taken up in dementia care to the same extent (or at least, the take-up has not been documented). Therefore, the aim of this chapter is to show the possibilities for providing reablement for individuals living with dementia. We will describe how individuals living with dementia can benefit from reablement and some of the possibilities and challenges in providing reablement to this user group.

This chapter begins with a short description of what dementia is and how the disease can impact on an individual's ability to participate in everyday living activities. We discuss how theoretical understandings of dementia developed in the late 20th century support a reablement approach to care for this population group. Dementia specific principles, techniques, and reablement intervention programs are presented to show that reablement in dementia care is possible and can be effective. Specifically, a literature search of published work regarding reablement intervention programs designed for individuals living with dementia was conducted, and readers are provided with examples of these intervention programs and descriptions of the impact these programs have had on individuals participating in them. Finally, the discussion is used to highlight some of the challenges in accessing reablement intervention programs for this population group.

Dementia interferes with an individual's ability to do everyday activities

Dementia is an umbrella term used to describe a collection of symptoms associated with multiple diseases impacting the brain (World Health Organization, 2012). It causes deterioration in thinking skills, sometimes referred to as 'cognitive abilities', which impacts on an individual's ability to participate in everyday tasks and be functionally independent (World Health Organization, 2012). While dementia is not a normal part of ageing, it primarily presents in individuals aged over 65 (Livingston et al, 2017). The most common cause of dementia is Alzheimer's disease (Burns and Iliffe, 2009). Other dementias include frontotemporal, Lewy body, vascular, and mixed dementia (Burns and Iliffe, 2009). A new case of dementia is diagnosed once every 3 seconds, which means that the number of individuals living with dementia worldwide is estimated to more than triple by 2050 (Alzheimer's Disease International, 2013; Prince et al, 2015) – although some research has found that the incidence of dementia may be declining in high-income countries (Prince et al, 2016; Taudorf et al, 2019). In 2018, around 50 million individuals worldwide lived with dementia (World Health Organization, 2020).

Common characteristics of any type of dementia include impairment in executive function, language, memory, perception, and changes in personality that impact on an individual's capability to participate in everyday living activities (Burns and Iliffe, 2009; Garcia-Alvarez et al, 2019). However, symptoms vary from individual to individual, and according to the type of dementia. There is no cure (Kenigsberg et al, 2016) and the loss of cognitive and physical function will eventually lead to death. Following a diagnosis, an individual typically lives around 7–10 years; some can live with dementia over 20 years (Fitzpatrick et al, 2005; Brodaty et al, 2012).

The progressive trajectory of dementia means that the condition will worsen over time and those who are impacted will eventually need help with all aspects of everyday life. The World Health Organization (WHO) has recognised dementia as a public health priority (2012). In 2017, the WHO global action plan on the public health response to dementia identified that individuals with dementia and their care partners should be offered interventions that enhance function and capability (World Health Organization, 2017).

Given the progressive nature of the disease, dementia can be classified in stages: mild, moderate, and severe (Dementia Australia, 2020). The progression through these stages can happen very fast (in a period of just a few months) or more slowly (over several years). The mild stage can sometimes be missed as the symptoms are less severe, and they have less impact on the individual's functional ability. However, as dementia progresses, an individual's ability to engage in everyday living activities as well as participate in family and community living is impacted (Dementia Australia, 2020). An individual typically first experiences difficulties, and requires support with instrumental activities of daily living (IADL; such as money management and shopping). Over time, they may require support with performing everyday living activities (ADL; such as grooming and bathing), all daily activities which are a focus in the reablement intervention. Other disabilities such as aphasia and other language and communication difficulties, visual and hearing difficulties (because dementia can impact parts of brain that process information coming from the eyes or ears), and changes in spatial and depth perception may also be experienced by individuals living with dementia. At the severe stage of the disease, the individual becomes increasingly disabled and will eventually need full-time care. The disabilities and reduced abilities to perform everyday living activities may also impact on an individual's roles within family and marriage. Feelings of being a burden are common and an individual's sense of self is impacted. Many individuals with dementia experience increased loneliness and isolation (Caddell and Clare, 2010).

Given reablement aims to address an individual's ability to participate in everyday living or social activities, it could be a helpful approach in enabling individuals with dementia to remain living at home and functionally independent (if they so wish) and engaged in their communities. More specifically, reablement interventions that adopt a philosophy around the possibilities that individuals have for living well with dementia, and what individuals with dementia can do given appropriate support, have the potential to assist this user group to engage in meaningful everyday living tasks and maintain or improve physical and psychosocial function as well as social participation (Clare, 2017; Poulos et al, 2017). The next section will discuss how the theoretical understandings of dementia, that developed in the late 20th century, have made reablement a possible approach to care for this user group.

New theories about dementia: opportunities for new therapeutic efforts

Theoretical assumptions are inherent in all interventions; they inform professional actions, whether they are explicated or not (Hammell, 2006; Thuesen et al, 2021). The theories underpinning reablement programmes may vary (see also Chapter 2 by Tuntland et al). Theories related to dementia may concern the conceptualisation of dementia (Downs et al, 2006), and disability (Shakespeare et al, 2017; Alzheimer Europe, 2018) both of which are described later. The conceptualisation of dementia, which we as individuals and societies adopt, will impact both how we support individuals and their families living with dementia as well as the experience of individuals living with dementia (Downs et al, 2006).

Theories about dementia have changed over time. Within western cultures, the dominant view on dementia has historically been the association of dementia with impaired cognitive functioning and as a normal and inevitable part of ageing (Downs et al, 2006). Yet, throughout most of the twentieth century a neuropsychiatric approach to understanding dementia has been more prevalent. This approach has conceptualised dementia as a progressive brain disease with biological deterioration. In the 1980s, a new understanding was introduced, explaining dementia as an interplay between neurological impairment and psychosocial factors – health, individual psychology and the environment, in particular the social context (Downs et al, 2006). This thinking has been ascribed to the British social psychologist Tom Kitwood, as quoted here by Linda Clare:

> The brain has considerable potential for change (plasticity), some of which is retained in dementia, and brain structure is shaped by a lifelong process of development in response to experience and environment. Psychological experience may affect brain structure just as brain structure may affect experience. While a malignant social environment might contribute to excess disability and speed up decline, Kitwood believed that a benign social psychology coupled with an enriched environment might facilitate some regeneration, or at least the maintenance of function for a period of time, and there is some evidence to support this. (Clare, 2008: 9)

Understanding dementia as an interplay between neurological impairment and psychosocial factors has had profound implications for therapeutic efforts in dementia care, such as reablement. Following these new understandings, new approaches were introduced. These new approaches have focused on supporting individuals with dementia and their family members (collectively referred to as 'dyads') to actively cope with dementia by maintaining selfhood and identity, ensuring a rich social environment and adopting a rehabilitative approach (Downs et al, 2006). These approaches mirror the current principles and components of reablement. By modifying their living environments and enabling individuals with dementia to participate in meaningful everyday living activities, and engage with their families and communities, reablement services may support individuals with dementia to maintain selfhood and identity (Clare, 2017).

More recently, dementia has been considered as a disability (Shakespeare et al, 2017; Alzheimer Europe, 2018; Devandas-Aguilar, 2019). A disability perspective supports a rights-based approach. The individual with dementia should be recognised as an equal citizen and rights holder (Alzheimer Europe, 2018). The United Nations Convention on the Rights of Persons with Disabilities (United Nations, 2006) outlines the right of individuals with disability to be able to attain and maintain maximum independence, with the assistance of comprehensive rehabilitation services (Article 26(1)), including reablement services.

Reablement in dementia care compared to standard reablement

In principle, reablement in dementia care has the same characteristics as reablement designed for individuals without dementia (Poulos et al, 2017).

Yet, within dementia care, reablement differs from standard reablement in several ways including: the care recipients, intervention end goals, processes, and the need for specific health professional skills (Beresford et al, 2019).

- *A dyadic focus is encouraged (where possible)*: Following the importance of the social environment as discussed, reablement focuses on the individual with dementia as well as their (informal) care partner (meaning 'dyads'; where possible), rather than the individual with dementia only (Poulos et al, 2017). There may also be an increased focus on addressing social (and physical) environmental factors (Jeon et al, 2018).
- *Balancing restorative and compensatory measures*: In the context of dementia, the purpose of reablement is to address the impact of cognitive impairment on everyday living activities. This includes the provision of support for an individual's physical function and mobility, cognition, communication, and social participation (Poulos et al, 2017). Here, restorative as well as compensatory measures are used (Clare, 2017).
- *Less focus on independence*: It should also be noted that while in the current definition of reablement (Metzelthin et al, 2020: 11) presented in Chapter 1 by Rostgaard et al, 'increasing or maintaining independence' is fundamental; yet such goals may not be achievable in dementia care. For example, in the context of dementia, expectations for regained independence may be inappropriate (Beresford et al, 2019) and goals of improving or maintaining function should only be applied when the care recipient identifies these as relevant and meaningful goals (Clare et al, 2019b). As such, individuals living with dementia who are unable to achieve independence-specific goals should not be excluded from reablement. Instead, accepting and adjusting to dementia diagnosis and maintaining social networks may be better suited reablement goals for individuals living with dementia (Beresford et al, 2019). Thus, pre-reablement processes and needs assessment are further stressed as crucial aspects of reablement in dementia care, and flexibility in practice (such as duration of home visits) should be incorporated into delivery models (Beresford et al, 2019).
- *Dementia-specific skills*: Finally, knowledge about dementia among health professionals who deliver care for individuals with dementia is important, not least when applying reablement. Communication skills, and the ability to teach and learn (reablement) intervention techniques are crucial for goal achievement and improved outcomes during reablement (Beresford et al, 2019; Jogie et al, 2021).

The next section provides an overview of effective reablement techniques that have been suggested for use in contemporary literature.

Suggested techniques for reablement in dementia care

Individuals with mild to moderate dementia have a relatively well-preserved ability for procedural learning often required in a reablement intervention. With appropriate support they can set and achieve goals, change behaviour, learn new ways of doing things, learn or relearn important information to improve functions in everyday life, and, if they are able and wish to, maintain independence in chosen activities (Clare et al 2019b; Jogie et al, 2021).

Systematic reviews of intervention programs that use reablement-type approaches for dementia show that functional decline associated with the disease can be delayed through tailored multi-component interventions (interventions that combine two or more treatment strategies) (McLaren et al, 2013; Scott et al, 2019). Slowing down functional decline means that individuals with dementia are more likely to be able to participate and complete everyday living activities for longer and require less help to remain living at home. Table 8.1 summarises techniques that can be adopted to support participation and activity engagement for individuals with dementia through reablement interventions. Interventions that improve the physical home environment (for example by including railing, adjusting lighting, or decluttering), the ability of the individual with dementia to participate in everyday living activities, and the knowledge and skills of their (informal) care partner, have been found to be the most effective in delaying functional decline associated with dementia (Laver, 2014).

In addition, of psychosocial interventions aimed at reducing behaviours of concern and psychological difficulties related to dementia, interventions that are comprised of multiple components over a set length of time and in the individual's home, have been shown to be most effective (Brodaty and Arasaratnam, 2012; Laver et al, 2014; Bennett et al, 2019; Livingston et al, 2020). These interventions are tailored to meet an individual's needs and engage informal care partners of the individual with dementia.

Identification of effective reablement intervention programs for individuals with dementia

While Table 8.1 provides an overview of available techniques, an aim of this chapter is also to identify reablement intervention programs which are available for individuals with dementia, and to consider their effectiveness. We sought to identify the extent and nature of available research pertaining to reablement intervention programs designed specifically for individuals with dementia (and their informal care partners). Our question was: what kind of programs are there for individuals with dementia, and what impact have these programs had on the participating individuals and their care partners?

Table 8.1: Techniques that can be adopted in reablement for individuals with dementia

Domain	Technique

Structuring the environment	• Using or adding cues that can help support independence. This could include using calendars, whiteboards with reminders, and/or clocks in open spaces to aide with planning for the day ahead.
	
	• Modifying the environment to ensure it is more enabling for the individual with dementia through:
	  · decluttering spaces
	  · using of appropriate lighting
	  · reducing noise
	  · modifying communication
	  · providing assistive technologies (such as personal alarm/falls monitor)
	  · making environmental modifications (such as clearly labelling cupboards, installing rails)

Structuring the activity	• Ensuring that activities are meaningful and produce value for the individual. This is best done through assessment of abilities and interests. • Practising everyday living activities to support continued everyday functioning. For example, a family member or home care provider may assist with putting on the washing machine, but the individual can finish the rest of the laundry task (hanging out, bringing in, folding, putting away). • Establishing and using strategies to compensate for functional changes. For example, using a timer when cooking or using a list when shopping.
Supporting the informal care partner (where possible)	• Highlighting the abilities of the individual with dementia. • Educating on dementia related topics including symptoms and associated changes. • Understanding the importance and impact of the home environment on everyday functioning. • Developing care partner skills such as strategies in problem solving, communication, activity simplification, and coping with stress. • Learning to identify changes in abilities and care situations as they arise, and generalising and adapting already learned skills to continue support participation. • Learning effective communication strategies, such as how to ask questions and provide instructions.

Source: Adapted from Poulos et al (2017)

Methodology

A search of published literature was completed to identify intervention programs that adopted the reablement approach described in this book (Metzelthin et al, 2020) and techniques consistent with this approach (such as those described in Table 8.1). The search strategy consisted of comprehensive searches of well-known databases including MEDLINE, PsycINFO, CINAHL, Cochrane Central Register of Controlled Trials, EMBASE, and Ageline, until September 2020. The strategies were used in earlier reviews (Ravn et al, 2019; Jogie et al, 2021) and combined terms relating to dementia, reablement (rehabilitation or restorative care) and community and/or residential aged care home services. To be considered for inclusion in this chapter, the studies had to be randomised controlled trials, non-randomised, or pre- and post-evaluation studies describing the impact of the intervention on everyday living activities (ADL), quality of life, behavioural changes related to dementia, and/or social participation.

Studies involving individuals living with dementia were included if the individual was participating in a reablement intervention program. As there is a well-documented terminological heterogeneity in this field (Clare, 2017), intervention programs may have been called rehabilitation, restorative care, or reablement in the original paper. The intervention program needed to consist of assessment, goal setting, several intervention sessions, and be delivered by an interdisciplinary team. The intervention also needed to focus on supporting an individual to achieve their goals, for example through participation in everyday living activities, physical activities, and/or exercise, home modifications, use of assistive technologies, and/or involvement of their social network.

Results

Six reablement intervention programs were identified. Four programs were delivered in the individual's home, and two in a residential aged care home. A summary of the characteristics of each is presented in Table 8.2 and each program is briefly described in the text that follows. A summary of common program characteristics is provided in the end.

The Care of Persons with Dementia in Their Environments

In the United States, the COPE intervention was designed to support everyday functioning of individuals with dementia, and the wellbeing of

Table 8.2: Reablement intervention programmes for individuals with dementia

Intervention program, author (year), country	Study design, target population, number of participants (n)	Health professional involved	Intervention duration and number of sessions	Reablement intervention components	Outcomes related to reablement intervention
COPE, Gitlin (2010), United States	RCT, mild to severe dementia, (MMSE 1–23), n = 237	Occupational therapist, nurse	Up to 4 months and 12 sessions with health professionals (10 sessions with an occupational therapist and 2 sessions with nurse).	Initial assessment of individual's abilities and deficits, home environment, care partner communication, and problems experienced by care partner. Care partner education and training to address self-identified areas of concerns. Review of care partner wellbeing and education around stress reduction. Care partner training in problem-solving, communication, engaging the individual with dementia in activities, and task simplification. Generalisation of knowledge and skills for future.	At 4 months, COPE participants showed less functional dependence and less dependence in IADLs compared with usual care participants; however, these were not observed long-term (at 9 months). Care partners showed better outcomes related to wellbeing, knowledge, and caregiving skills compared with care partners in usual care group at both short and long-term.
GREAT, Clare et al (2013, 2019a, 2019b), United Kingdom	RCT, AD, vascular or mixed dementia, or mild-to-moderate cognitive impairment as indicated by a MMSE score ≥18, n = 475	Occupational therapist or nurse; could be other health professional trained in intervention	Total 9 months with weekly sessions over up to 3 months and maintenance sessions for subsequent 6 months. Ten weekly 1-hour individual sessions followed by four 1-hour maintenance sessions.	Participants choose rehabilitation goals, and these are addressed in subsequent sessions. Strategies and education around difficulties experienced with emotion regulation and behavioural activation; reviewing and adjusting the use of strategies to address areas of concern, identifying and educating about other relevant services and supports, and care partner support.	At 3 months, there were statistically significant large positive effects for participant-rated goal attainment at 3 months and these effects were maintained at 9 months (corroborated by care partner ratings). No significant change in quality of life at 3 or 9 months.

(continued)

Table 8.2: Reablement intervention programmes for individuals with dementia (continued)

Intervention program, author (year), country	Study design, target population, number of participants (n)	Health professional involved	Intervention duration and number of sessions	Reablement intervention components	Outcomes related to reablement intervention
I-HARP Jeon et al (2019), Australia	RCT, aMCI or early/moderate stage dementia, n = 19	Occupational therapist, nurse, psychologist	Up to 4 months. Up to 12 home visits (~90 mins each).	Home visits from a member of multidisciplinary team (MDT) tailored to client's needs and care partner support needs. Up to A$1,000 (€630) towards assistive devices and environmental modifications. Begins with a comprehensive assessment including home environment, and review of their medication, cognitive and communication needs.	Short-term improvements in functional independence and QOL for individuals with dementia, and improved wellbeing for care partners. Longer-term slowing down of functional decline for the individuals with dementia and maintaining QOL of both individuals with dementia and care partner.
Home care assistance program Carbone et al (2013), Italy	Pre- and post- evaluation, mild to moderate AD, n = 22	MDT (nurses, occupational therapists, psychologists, and social assistants)	3 months, 6-hour sessions, three times per week.	Home visits from a member of MDT following comprehensive assessment of the individual's cognitive and behavioural capacities, functional and motor abilities, environmental and social situation, and care partner burden. Goals are set and reviewed monthly by the team. Activities focus on maintaining functional abilities such as ADLs and improving behavioural symptoms and cognitive capabilities. Psychological support and education are included, as well as occupational therapy to address needs around environmental modification and assistive devices.	Participants showed significant improvement regarding ADLs and behavioural changes related to dementia immediately following completion of intervention. However, these were not sustained long-term.

Table 8.2: Reablement intervention programmes for individuals with dementia (continued)

Intervention program, author (year), country	Study design, target population, number of participants (n)	Health professional involved	Intervention duration and number of sessions	Reablement intervention components	Outcomes related to reablement intervention
Lifeful, Low et al (2018), Australia	Pre- and post-evaluation, anyone in residential aged care facility (with focus on dementia), n = 80	All staff in the participating residential aged care facility	12 months, ongoing interaction in care facility.	Upskilling of staff (for example education regarding reablement approaches, activity engagement, and communication with individuals with dementia); Supporting organisational change through dedicated rostering, assigning residents a 'focus' care partner and focusing on the psychosocial care of residents ('all about me' with residents to understand their social and activity needs and to set goals, 'resident of the week' handovers, 3 monthly staff training.	Residents showed improvements in depressive symptoms, functioning, safety, activity engagement, dignity and overall QOL at 12 months.
FFC-CI, Galik et al (2013), United States	RCT, cognitively impaired residents (MMSE ≤15), n = 103	Nurse coordination. All staff involvement	6 months, 10 hours per week spent in each facility.	Begins with facility policy assessment and environmental evaluation to ensure suitability of intervention within facility and to determine possible barriers. Staff and family care partners are provided with education about FFC. Residents are engaged in identification and development of individualised goals. Facility care staff are engaged in ongoing education and mentoring related to how to provide FFC.	For individuals in intervention group: agitated behaviours and function improved at 3-months. Physical activity and activity engagement improved at 6-months.

Note: Abbreviations used: AD = Alzheimer's disease; ADL = Activities of daily living; aMCI = amnestic mild cognitive impairment; COPE = Care of Persons with dementia in their Environment; FFC-CI = Function-Focused Care for the Cognitively Impaired; GREAT = Goal-oriented cognitive rehabilitation; I-HARP = Interdisciplinary Home-bAsed Reablement Program; MDT = Multidisciplinary team; MMSE = Mini Mental Status Examination; QOL = Quality of Life; RACF = Residential aged care facility; RCT = Randomised controlled trial their care partner (Gitlin et al, 2010). The COPE intervention program consists of several fundamental elements of reablement, including improving physical health and function, engaging the individual in everyday activities, maintaining quality of life, and supporting care partners. It uses a multidisciplinary approach to care, and combined occupational therapy knowledge and skills together with nursing skills for management of medical symptoms and concerns. In the study by Gitlin and colleagues (2010), an occupational therapist visited the individual with dementia in their home for up to ten times over a period of (up to) 4 months. A systematic approach to care was used where the therapist worked collaboratively with the care partner to identify areas of concern. Care partners were then educated to problem solve different approaches around modifying their communication, the home environment and steps to encourage participation in activities of daily living. The therapist also educated the care partner about how to engage the individual in enjoyable activities based on their level of cognitive and functional ability. A nurse was involved for reviewing health needs and providing support for medications, hydration, continence, pain, and infection management (Gitlin et al, 2010). A randomised controlled study of over 200 individuals living with dementia and their care partners found improvements in the functional independence and participation in ADLs of COPE participants living with dementia at 4 months and in the wellbeing of their care partner at 4 and 9 months (Gitlin et al, 2010).

In 2016, the COPE intervention program was also adapted for use and implemented in Australia (Clemson et al, 2018; Clemson et al, 2020). One-hundred and four dyads participated in the Australian study, which also showed increased engagement in activities following participation in COPE for the individual with dementia and improved wellbeing and confidence in continuing to provide care at home for care partners (Clemson et al, 2020; Rahja et al, 2020b). As part of the implementation evaluation in Australia, a qualitative study with ten participant dyads was completed to learn about their experiences with COPE (Rahja et al, 2020a). This study described how the informal care partners felt that COPE's collaborative approach to care was 'empowering' as it helped them feel that they were able to continue to provide care at home for the individual living with dementia through learning stress management and problem-solving strategies around they key challenges they had identified (Rahja et al, 2020a). A powerful message from the individuals living with dementia and their care partners was also that that COPE had given them 'a second chance' to remain living at home and continue to participate in their chosen and valued roles and activities (Rahja et al, 2020a).

Goal-oriented cognitive rehabilitation (GREAT trial)

In the United Kingdom, a goal-oriented cognitive rehabilitation intervention for early-stage Alzheimer's and related dementias was evaluated in the GREAT trial (Clare et al, 2019a; Clare et al, 2019b). A randomised controlled study with 475 participants with dementia and mild to moderate cognitive impairment from eight different National Health Service (NHS) centres was conducted within the GREAT trial. The study found that individuals living with dementia and their care partners are able to identify and set goals to improve their everyday functioning using a goal setting tool (Bangor Goal Setting Interview – BGSI) (Clare et al, 2019b). The BGSI was developed using the Canadian Occupational Performance Measure (COPM) which is described in more detail in Chapter 6 by Tuntland et al. It consists of a structured format for determining individual goals in a way that enables goal attainment and progress over time to be measured in relation to each of the identified goals. The study showed significant effects in goal attainment for both individuals with dementia and their care partners at 3 and 9 months. The intervention was also found to be effective in improving everyday functioning in the specific areas identified through goal-setting at 3 months, and this improvement was maintained at 9 months (Clare et al, 2019a).

The intervention consisted of ten weekly home visits (over approximately 3 months) by a specially trained health professional. The individual with dementia and their informal care partner worked with the trained health professional who facilitated goal setting and the implementation of strategies that enabled the individual to work towards these goals. The goals addressed areas related to everyday function and social participation (Clare et al, 2019b). Other difficulties experienced by the individual with dementia were addressed through applying relevant strategies (such as emotion regulation), reviewing and adjusting their current use of strategies, providing support and opportunities to practice different strategies to address areas of concern, identifying and educating about other relevant services and supports, and offering support for care partners.

A subsequent study described experiences of participants (individuals with dementia and their informal care partners) in the GREAT study (Warmoth et al, 2020). Twenty-five individuals with mild dementia were interviewed and they described how they felt that, through the intervention program, their therapist had learned to understand the difficulties they experienced with everyday living with dementia, and their overall preferences for care. These participants talked about the importance of the relational nature of care they received. Through setting and achieving goals, the participants living with dementia described feeling enjoyment and empowerment. The informal care partners described that the individualised and tailored approach to care and the ongoing relationship with the therapist provided them increased confidence in problem-solving strategies and finding solutions (Warmoth et al, 2020). It was noted in this study that some informal care partners were unsure of the long-term benefits of the intervention, and not everyone considered reablement relevant (Warmoth et al, 2020).

Interdisciplinary Home-Based Reablement Program

The I-HARP program was designed in Australia to address the needs of individuals living with dementia and amnestic mild cognitive impairment (aMCI) (Jeon et al, 2017a; Jeon et al, 2017b; Jeon et al, 2020). The intervention was adapted from a reablement intervention aimed to reduce disability in cognitively intact older adults (Szanton et al, 2011; Szanton et al, 2014). A pilot randomised controlled study (with 18 participants) was completed to determine the potential impact of I-HARP on the participants' everyday living activities, mobility, quality of life, and mood, as well as care partner burden and quality of life (Jeon et al, 2020).

I-HARP consisted of up to 12 home visits (approximately 90 minutes each) from a member of the multidisciplinary team (occupational therapist, nurse, and psychologist). The visits were tailored to the client's and care partners' needs. Up to A$1,000 (€630) was afforded towards assistive devices and minor environmental modifications at an individual's home (such as installation of rails). The intervention continued for up to 4 months and began with a comprehensive assessment which was completed with the individual and their care partner. A review of their medication, cognitive, and communication needs was also completed, and goal setting was used to develop an individualised plan to address the individual's needs. I-HARP consisted of task simplification strategies, physical exercises, pain and/or mood management, problem solving, and medication education, as needed by directly addressing these abilities and factors (Jeon et al, 2019). An informal care partner was provided with individualised support, including practical strategies to address cognitive, functional, and psychosocial changes or other difficulties caused by the disease progression, education around dementia, and connecting them with services in the community following intervention completion (Jeon et al, 2020).

The initial results from the pilot study showed improvements in functional independence and quality of life for individuals with dementia, slowing down of functional decline, and improved care partner quality of life (Jeon et al, 2020). Interviews with care partners of individuals with dementia who took part in the pilot described how I-HARP had helped them better understand dementia, learn about how to manage behaviours of concern, and access supports or services (Jeon et al, 2020).

Home care assistance program

In Italy, a small (22 participants) pre- and post-evaluation was completed of a home care assistance program delivered by a multidisciplinary team for individuals with mild-to-moderate Alzheimer's type dementia (Carbone et al, 2013). The intervention lasted for up to 3 months and consisted of three sessions a week, lasting for 6 hours each. The intervention began with an assessment completed by a team of nurses, occupational therapists, psychologists, and social assistants. The assessment consisted of evaluation of the individual's cognitive and behavioural capabilities, functional and motor abilities, environmental and social situation, and care partner burden. Following assessment, goals were set, and these were reviewed in monthly team meetings. The intervention activities aimed to motivate participants to maintain their functional abilities, address behavioural changes related to dementia, and improve their cognitive capabilities. Psychological support and education around how to seek dementia specific support was also provided. An occupational therapist offered advice related to environmental modification and assistive devices. The intervention was found to improve participation in everyday living activities and behavioural changes related to dementia (Carbone et al, 2013).

LifeFul

The Australian LifeFul was designed to enable residential aged care facility staff to better engage with residents (Low et al, 2018). LifeFul was a 12-month intervention that aimed to equip staff to be more individualised and enabling in their attitude towards residents with dementia during social, physical, recreational, and other everyday activities. Each resident was allocated a 'focus carer' and the intervention consisted of implementing dedicated rostering, discussing reablement approaches during handovers, and supporting care facility managers in changing organisation policies and practices to support LifeFul. Regular staff training around communication and activity engagement strategies, incidental exercise, quality of life, and reablement approaches was also provided. A pre- and post-evaluation with 69 residents showed improvements in depressive symptoms, functioning, safety, activity engagement, dignity, and overall quality of life for residents following participation in LifeFul (Low et al, 2018).

Function-Focused Care for the Cognitively Impaired

In the United States, Function-Focused Care for the Cognitively Impaired (FFC-CI) was evaluated in a cluster randomised control study with individuals with dementia living in residential care (Galik et al, 2013).

The FFC-CI intervention lasted for 6 months during which the nurse engaged with each participating facility for 10 hours per week. The FFC-CI taught and mentored care facility staff to actively engage residents with cognitive impairment in individualised functional and physical activities. A nurse coordinated the delivery of the intervention, which was completed by other facility staff members. The intervention was divided into four components: 1) facility specific policy assessment and evaluation of the care facility environment to identify potential barriers for the intervention implementation in the facility; 2) family and staff education about function focused care; 3) identification and development of individualised goals in collaboration with the resident, nurse, family, and staff; and 4) dedicated FFC-CI 'champions' and provision of ongoing education and mentoring of staff by the FFC Nurse and facility champions (Galik et al, 2013).

A 6-month evaluation with 103 residents with dementia showed significant improvements in outcomes relating to physical activity and activity engagement for participants in the FFC-CI intervention group (Galik et al, 2013).

Summary of common features across reablement intervention programs in dementia care

To summarise, there are only a few studies describing reablement interventions programs designed specifically for individuals with dementia that have been evaluated in research studies.

Of the programs that were provided in the community, all engaged at least occupational therapists and nurses. Other common features of the included programs were the 3–4-month duration which included weekly sessions with healthcare professionals. All programs also began with comprehensive assessment and goal setting which guided the individualised intervention plan and included care partner engagement. In addition, all programs had a focus on the individual to be able to continue participation in everyday living and/or other meaningful activities and had a focus on evaluating and ensuring that the individual's living environment provided opportunities for activity engagement. Most programs also provided additional focus on changes in behaviours that the individual with dementia was experiencing/ having difficulty with.

Programs in residential aged care homes were less common. The included programs had similarities in that both engaged in care home specific environmental and policy assessment to support reablement approaches, staff training and engaging informal care partners and encouraging participation in everyday living activities. Similar features have been described in more recent research studies of reablement programs in residential aged care homes which have yielded similar, positive, outcomes related to activity engagement and quality of life for residents (Galik et al, 2021; Yang et al, 2021).

The reablement programs that have been described in research studies have shown promising results in terms of enabling individuals with dementia to engage in meaningful everyday living activities. These programs have supported informal care partners to feel empowered to continue providing care at home through learning strategies around stress management, problem solving, and finding strategies around key challenges. Underpinning these findings was the reablement focus on identifying the individual's capabilities and using these capabilities to engage the individual in everyday living activities.

Discussion: challenges of reablement in dementia care

This chapter has described how reablement is a worthy approach and practice in dementia care. Several techniques and intervention programs have been described that can be used in practice. Yet, despite the potential benefits of reablement interventions for individuals living with dementia, reablement has not been integrated in dementia research and/or care in the same way as it has been in usual aged care. As such, there is a lack of strong research evidence to support this approach, which may be because individuals with dementia are often excluded from research studies. Within clinical practice, barriers to accessing reablement intervention programs for individuals with dementia also exist, and just a few of these are outlined in the following paragraphs.

Stigma towards individuals living with dementia is well-documented among the general public, family members, and health professionals (Werner and Giveon, 2008; Batsch and Mittelman, 2012; Mukadam and Livingston, 2012; Dementia Australia, 2017; Herrmann et al, 2018). Many health professionals believe that nothing can be done to help individuals living with dementia (Batsch and Mittelman, 2012; Goodwin and Allan, 2018). For example, in Australia, interviews with healthcare professionals working in rehabilitation settings have revealed that interventions for individuals with dementia are seldom considered as worthy of the investment of limited resources (such as time or money) and many have questioned that individuals with dementia could benefit from interventions that are restorative and provide meaningful outcomes (Cations et al, 2020).

This chapter has also outlined that reablement interventions to support individuals with dementia require specialist dementia knowledge. However, dementia education among health professionals varies. Training of the dementia workforce in evidence-based interventions is limited (Hodgson and Gitlin, 2021) and healthcare professionals have shown limited understanding of the pathology of the disease and its progression (Hsu et al, 2005; Smyth et al, 2013; Robinson et al, 2014). This leads to lack of readiness to work with individuals with dementia (Hsu et al, 2005). An additional challenge to accessing reablement may be the availability of the health–related services to individuals with dementia in a given country. For example, in Australia, individuals with dementia who live in the community may need to wait up to 2 years or longer to be able to access services that adopt a reablement approach (Department of Health, 2020) and such services are also rarely available. In Denmark, reablement was introduced by law in 2015 (see Chapter 9 by Rostgaard and Graff), and the law text includes older people living with dementia as a target group. Yet, it is not known to what extent individuals with dementia are included in regular reablement intervention programs. Research suggests that individuals with dementia may more often be provided with care that incorporates a reabling mindset rather than being included in regular reablement intervention programs (Thuesen, 2021; Graff et al, 2022). Similar challenges to accessibility and availability of reablement services directed to individuals with dementia can been seen across the globe.

Delays in dementia diagnosis can also hinder access to reablement programs for this population group. While general practitioners (also known as family doctors, medical practitioners, or general physicians) are in key position to identify symptoms, diagnose, and organise specialist dementia supports (Speechly et al, 2008; Iliffe et al, 2009; Ng and Ward, 2019), they may be hesitant to suggest dementia as a possible diagnosis due to their limited knowledge about the disease (Iliffe et al, 2003; Smyth et al, 2013; Robinson et al, 2014; Ng and Ward, 2019). Some general practitioners also believe that diagnosis would not change patient care management (van Hout et al, 2007; Ahmad et al, 2010). Yet, while specialists are more confident in diagnosing dementia compared with general practitioners, depending on the country and its health care system, they can be expensive and difficult to access. Finally, formal supports for dementia are most often sought at a point of crises, such as during hospitalisation following an illness or injury (Vroomen et al, 2013). As such, opportunities to access preventative interventions, such as reablement, are reduced, as care is not accessed at the time of initial symptom presentation or dementia diagnosis.

Conclusion

This chapter has illustrated that there is promise for reablement in dementia care. Theories are presented that are currently used to describe dementia and how they provide an opportunity to consider a reablement approach to care for this population group. This chapter has described how reablement in dementia care differs from reablement in standard care and has provided readers with reablement techniques that can be used when working with individuals with dementia. Through a literature search, reablement intervention programs have been identified that have been evaluated in research studies and key reablement characteristics have been summarised that were prevalent in these programs. While reablement is more commonly used in the community, it can also be used in residential aged care homes, although this may more likely require an organisational approach and review of current care home practices. Regardless of the setting where reablement is provided, possible benefits for individuals with dementia from taking part in these intervention programs are shown. Finally, the chapter has discussed why reablement has not been integrated in dementia care to the same extent as it has been in usual aged care. Some of the challenges for this are stigma towards individuals living with dementia, lack of formal health professional education in reablement for this population group, and delayed diagnosis, which hinders opportunities for early intervention.

References

Ahmad, S., Orrell, M., Iliffe, S., and Gracie, A. (2010) 'GPs' attitudes, awareness, and practice regarding early diagnosis of dementia', *The British Journal of General Practice*, 60: e360–e5.

Alzheimer Europe (2018) '2017: Dementia as a disability? Implications for ethics, policy and practice', [online], Available from: https://www.alzhei mer-europe.org/Ethics/Ethical-issues-in-practice/2017-Dementia-as-a-dis ability-Implications-for-ethics-policy-and-practice/Human-rights-and-opportunities.

Alzheimer's Disease International (2013) *Policy Brief for G8 Heads of Government: The Global Impact of Dementia 2013–2050*, London: Alzheimer's Disease International (ADI).

Batsch, N. and Mittelman, M. (2012) *World Alzheimer Report 2012. Overcoming the Stigma of Dementia*, London, UK: Alzheimer's Disease International (ADI).

Bennett, S., Laver, K., Voigt-Radloff, S., Letts, L., Clemson, L., Graff, M., Wiseman, J., and Gitlin, L. (2019) 'Occupational therapy for people with dementia and their family carers provided at home: a systematic review and meta-analysis', *BMJ Open*, 9: e026308.

Beresford, B., Mann, R., Parker, G., Kanaan, M., Faria, R., Rabiee, P., Weatherly, H., Clarke, S., Mayhew, E., Duarte, A., Laver-Fawcett, A., and Aspinal, F. (2019) 'Reablement services for people at risk of needing social care: the MoRe mixed-methods evaluation', *Health Services and Delivery Research*, 7: 1–218.

Brodaty, H. and Arasaratnam, C. (2012) 'Meta-analysis of nonpharmacological interventions for neuropsychiatric symptoms of dementia', *American Journal of Psychiatry*, 169: 946–53.

Brodaty, H., Seeher, K., and Gibson, L. (2012) 'Dementia time to death: a systematic literature review on survival time and years of life lost in people with dementia', *International Psychogeriatrics*, 24: 1034–45.

Burns, A. and Iliffe, S. (2009) 'Dementia', *BMJ*, 338: b75.

Caddell, L. and Clare, L. (2010) 'The impact of dementia on self and identity: a systematic review', *Clinical Psychology Review*, 30: 113–26.

Carbone, G., Barreca, F., Mancini, G., Pauletti, G., Salvi, V., Vanacore, N., Salvitti, C., Ubaldi, F., and Sinibaldi, L. (2013) 'A home assistance model for dementia: outcome in patients with mild-to-moderate Alzheimer's disease after three months', *Annali dell'Istituto Superiore di Sanita*, 49: 34–41.

Cations, M., May, N., Whitehead, C., Crotty, M., Clemson, L., Low, L.-F., Mcloughlin, J., Swaffer, K., and Laver, K.E. (2020) 'Health professional perspectives on rehabilitation for people with dementia', *The Gerontologist*, 60(3): 503–12.

Clare, L. (2008) *Neuropsychological Rehabilitation and People with Dementia*, New York: Psychology Press.

Clare, L. (2017) 'Rehabilitation for people living with dementia: a practical framework of positive support', *PLoS Medicine*, 14: e1002245.

Clare, L., Bayer, A., Burns, A., Corbett, A., Jones, R., Knapp, M., Kopelmann, M., Kudlicka A., Iracema, L., Oyebode, J., Woods, B., and Whitaker, R. (2013) 'Goal-oriented cognitive rehabilitation in early-stage dementia: study protocol for a multi-centre single-blind randomised controlled trial (GREAT)', *Trials*, 14: 152.

Clare, L., Kudlicka, A., Oyebode, J., Jones, R., Bayer, A., Leroi, I., Kopelman, M., James, I., Culverwell, A., Pool, J., Brand, A., Henderson, C., Hoare, Z., Knapp, M., and Woods, B. (2019a) 'Individual goal-oriented cognitive rehabilitation to improve everyday functioning for people with early-stage dementia: a multicentre randomised controlled trial (the GREAT trial)', *International Journal of Geriatric Psychiatry*, 34(5): 709–21.

Clare, L., Kudlicka, A., Oyebode, J., Jones, R., Bayer, A., Leroi, I., Kopelman, M., James, I., Culverwell, A., Pool, J., Brand, A., Henderson, C., Hoare, Z., Knapp, M., Morgan-Trimmer, S., Burns, A., Corbett, A., Whitaker, R., and Woods, B. (2019b) 'Goal-oriented cognitive rehabilitation for early-stage Alzheimer's and related dementias: the GREAT RCT', *Health Technology Assessment*, 23:709–21.

Clemson, L., Laver, K., Jeon, Y.-H., Comans, T., Scanlan, J., Rahja, M., Culph, J., Low, L.-F., Day, S., Cations, M., Crotty, M., Kurrle, S., Piersol, C., and Gitlin, L. (2018) 'Implementation of an evidence-based intervention to improve the wellbeing of people with dementia and their carers: study protocol for "Care of People with dementia in their Environments (COPE)" in the Australian context', *BMC Geriatrics*, 18: 108.

Clemson, L., Laver, K., Rahja, M., Culph, J., Scanlan, J., Day, S., Comans, T., Jeon, Y.-H., Low, L.-F., Crotty, M., Kurrle, S., Cations, M., Piersol, C., and Gitlin, L. (2020) 'Implementing a reablement intervention, "Care of People with dementia in their Environments (COPE)": a hybrid implementation-effectiveness study', *The Gerontologist*, 61(6): 965–76.

Dementia Australia (2017) 'Dementia and the impact of stigma', [online], Available from: https://www.dementia.org.au/sites/default/files/NATIONAL/documents/dementia-and-stigma-2017.pdf

Dementia Australia (2020) 'Progression of dementia' [online], Available from: https://www.dementia.org.au/about-dementia/what-is-dementia/progression-of-dementia

Department of Health (2020) *Home Care Packages Program: Data Report 1st Quarter 2020–21*. Canberra [online], Available from: https://www.gen-agedcaredata.gov.au/www_aihwgen/media/Home_care_report/HCPP-Data-Report-2020-2021-1st-qtr.pdf

Devandas-Aguilar, C. (2019) *Report of the Special Rapporteur on the Rights of Persons with Disabilities*. Seventy-Fourth Session, United Nations.

Downs, M., Clare, L., and Mackenzie, J. (2006) 'Understandings of dementia: explanatory models and their implications for the person with dementia and therapeutic effort' in J.C. Hughes, S.J. Louw, and S.R. Sabat (eds) *Dementia: Mind, Meaning and the Person*, Oxford: Oxford University Press.

Fitzpatrick, A., Kuller, L., Lopez, O., Kawas, C., and Jagust, W. (2005) 'Survival following dementia onset: Alzheimer's disease and vascular dementia', *Journal of the Neurological Sciences*, 229–30: 43–9.

Galik, E.M., Resnick, B., Hammersla, M., and Brightwater, J. (2013) 'Optimizing function and physical activity among nursing home residents with dementia: testing the impact of function-focused care', *The Gerontologist*, 54: 930–43.

Galik, E.M., Resnick, B., Holmes, S.D., Vigne, E., Lynch, K., Ellis, J., and Barr, E. (2021) 'A cluster randomized controlled trial testing the impact of function and behavior focused care for nursing home residents with dementia', *Journal of the American Medical Directors Association*, 22(7): 1421–88.e4.

Garcia-Alvarez, L., Gomar, J., Sousa, A., Garcia-Portilla, M., and Goldberg, T. (2019) 'Breadth and depth of working memory and executive function compromises in mild cognitive impairment and their relationships to frontal lobe morphometry and functional competence', *Alzheimer's & Dementia: Diagnosis, Assessment & Disease Monitoring*, 11: 170–9.

Gitlin, L., Winter, L., Dennis, M., Hodgson, N., and Hauck, W. (2010) 'A biobehavioral home-based intervention and the well-being of patients with dementia and their caregivers: the COPE randomized trial', *Journal of American Medical Association*, 304: 983–91.

Goodwin, V. and Allan, L. (2018) '"Mrs Smith has no rehab potential": does rehabilitation have a role in the management of people with dementia?', *Age and Ageing*, 48: 5–7.

Graff, L., Timm, H., and Thuesen, J. (forthcoming) 'Organizational narratives in rehabilitation-focused dementia care – negotiating identities, interventions and personhood', *Dementia*.

Hammell, K. (2006) *Perspectives on Disability and Rehabilitation: Contesting Assumptions, Challenging Practice*, London: Elsevier Health Sciences.

Herrmann, L., Welter, E., Leverenz, J., Lerner, A.J., Udelson, N., Kanetsky, C., and Sajatovic, M. (2018) 'A systematic review of dementia-related stigma research: can we move the stigma dial?', *The American Journal of Geriatric Psychiatry*, 26: 316–31.

Hodgson, N. and Gitlin, L. (2021) 'Implementing and sustaining family care programs in real world settings: barriers and facilitators', in J.E. Gaugler (ed) *Bridging the Family Care Gap*, London: Elsevier.

Hsu, M.C., Moyle, W., Creedy, D., and Venturato, L. (2005) 'An investigation of aged care mental health knowledge of Queensland aged care nurses', *International Journal of Mental Health Nursing*, 14: 16–23.

Iliffe, S., Manthorpe, J., and Eden, A. (2003) 'Sooner or later? Issues in the early diagnosis of dementia in general practice: a qualitative study', *Family Practice*, 20: 376–81.

Iliffe, S., Robinson, L., Brayne, C., Goodman, C., Rait, G., Manthorpe, J., and Ashley, P. (2009) 'Primary care and dementia: 1. Diagnosis, screening and disclosure', *International Journal of Geriatric Psychiatry*, 24: 895–901.

Jeon, Y.-H., Clemson, L., Naismith, S., Mowszowski, L., Mcdonagh, N., Mackenzie, M., Dawes, C., Krein, L., and Szanton, S.L. (2017a) 'Improving the social health of community-dwelling older people living with dementia through a reablement program', *International Psychogeriatrics*, 30(6): 915–20.

Jeon, Y.-H., Clemson, L., Naismith, S., Szanton, S.L., Simpson, J.M., Low, L.-F., Mowszowski, L., Gonski, P., Norman, R., Krein, L., Gitlin, L., and Brodaty, H. (2017b) 'Optimising independence of older persons with cognitive and functional decline: interdisciplinary home-based reablement program (I-HARP)', *Alzheimer's & Dementia: The Journal of the Alzheimer's Association*, 13: P1157.

Jeon, Y.-H., Clemson, L., Naismith, S., Mowszowski, L., Mcdonagh, N., Mackenzie, M., Dawes, C., Krein, L., and Szanton, S.L. (2018) 'Improving the social health of community-dwelling older people living with dementia through a reablement program', *International Psychogeriatrics*, 30: 915–20.

Jeon, Y.-H., Simpson, J., Low, L.-F., Woods, R., Norman, R., Mowszowski, L., Clemson, L., Naismith, S., Brodaty, H., Hilmer, S.N., Amberber, A., Gitlin, L., and Szanton, S.L. (2019) 'A pragmatic randomised controlled trial (RCT) and realist evaluation of the interdisciplinary home-bAsed Reablement program (I-HARP) for improving functional independence of community dwelling older people with dementia: an effectiveness-implementation hybrid design', *BMC Geriatrics*, 19: 199.

Jeon, Y.-H., Krein, L., Simpson, J., Szanton, S.L., Clemson, L., Naismith, S., Low, L.-F., Mowszowski, L., Gonski, P., Norman, R., Gitlin, L., and Brodaty, H. (2020) 'Feasibility and potential effects of interdisciplinary home-based reablement program (I-HARP) for people with cognitive and functional decline: A pilot trial', *Aging & Mental Health*, 24: 1916–25.

Jogie, P., Rahja, M., Van Den Berg, M., Cations, M., Brown, S., and Laver, K. (2021) 'Goal setting for people with mild cognitive impairment or dementia in rehabilitation: a scoping review', *Australian Occupational Therapy Journal*, 68(6): 563–92.

Kenigsberg, P.A., Aquino, J.P., Berard, A., Gzil, F., Andrieu, S., Banerjee, S., Bremond, F., Buee, L., Cohen-Mansfield, J., Mangialasche, F., Platel, H., Salmon, E., and Robert, P. (2016) 'Dementia beyond 2025: knowledge and uncertainties', *Dementia*, 15: 6–21.

Laver, K., Clemson, L., Bennett, S., Lannin, N., and Brodaty, H. (2014) 'Unpacking the evidence: interventions for reducing behavioral and psychological symptoms in people with dementia', *Physical & Occupational Therapy in Geriatrics*, 32: 294–309.

Livingston, G., Sommerlad, A., Orgeta, V., Costafreda, S.G., Huntley, J., Ames, D., Ballard, C., Banerjee, S., Burns, A., Cohen-Mansfield, J., Cooper, C., Fox, N., Gitlin, L., Howard, R., Kales, H.C., Larson, E.B., Ritchie, K., Rockwood, K., Sampson, E.L., Samus, Q., Schneider, L.S., Selbaek, G., Teri, L., and Mukadam, N. (2017) 'Dementia prevention, intervention, and care', *Lancet*, 390: 2673–734.

Livingston, G., Huntley, J., Sommerlad, A., Ames, D., Ballard, C., Banerjee, S., Brayne, C., Burns, A., Cohen-Mansfield, J., Cooper, C., Costafreda, S., Dias, A., Fox, N., Gitlin, L., Howard, R., Kales, H., Kivimäki, M., Larson, E., Ogunniyi, A., Orgeta, V., Ritchie, K., Rockwood, K., Sampson, E., Samus, Q., Schneider, L., Selbæk, G., Teri, L., and Mukadam, N. (2020) 'Dementia prevention, intervention, and care: 2020 report of the *Lancet* Commission', *Lancet*, 396: 413–46.

Low, L.-F., Venkatesh, S., Clemson, L., Merom, D., Casey, A.-N., and Brodaty, H. (2018) 'Feasibility of LifeFul: a relationship and reablement-focused culture change program in residential aged care', *BMC Geriatrics*, 18: 129.

Mclaren, A.N., Lamantia, C.M., and Callahan, M. (2013) 'Systematic review of non-pharmacologic interventions to delay functional decline in community-dwelling patients with dementia', *Aging & Mental Health*, 17: 655–66.

Metzelthin, S., Rostgaard, T., Parsons, M., and Burton, E. (2020) 'Development of an internationally accepted definition of reablement: a Delphi study', *Ageing and Society*, 42(3): 703–18.

Mukadam, N. and Livingston, G. (2012) 'Reducing the stigma associated with dementia: approaches and goals', *Aging Health*, 8: 377–86.

Ng, N.S.Q. and Ward, S.A. (2019) 'Diagnosis of dementia in Australia: a narrative review of services and models of care', *Australian Health Review*, 43: 415–24.

Poulos, C., Bayer, A., Beaupre, L.A., Clare, L., Poulos, R.G., Wang, R.H., Zuidema, S.U., and Mcgilton, K. (2017) 'A comprehensive approach to reablement in dementia', *Alzheimer's & Dementia*, 3: 450–8.

Prince, M., Wimo, A., Guerchet, M., Ali, G.-C., Wu, Y.-T., Prina, M., Chan, K.Y., Xia, Z., and Alzheimer's Disease International (2015) *World Alzheimer Report 2015. The Global Impact of Dementia: An Analysis of Prevalence, Incidence, Cost and Trends*, London: Alzheimer's Disease International (ADI).

Prince, M., Ali, G.C., Guerchet, M., Prina, A.M., Albanese, E., and Wu, Y.T. (2016) 'Recent global trends in the prevalence and incidence of dementia, and survival with dementia', *Alzheimer's Research & Therapy*, 8: 23.

Rahja, M., Culph, J., Clemson, L., Day, S., and Laver, K. (2020a) 'A second chance: Experiences and outcomes of people with dementia and their families participating in a dementia reablement program', *Brain Impairment*, 21(3): 274–85.

Rahja, M., Nguyen, K.-H., Laver, K., Clemson, L., Crotty, M., and Comans, T. (2020b) 'Implementing an evidence-based dementia care program in the Australian health context: a cost–benefit analysis', *Health & Social Care in the Community*, 28: 2013–24.

Ravn, M.B., Petersen, K.S., and Thuesen, J. (2019) 'Rehabilitation for people living with dementia: a scoping review of processes and outcomes', *Journal of Aging Research*: 4141050.

Robinson, A., Eccleston, C., Annear, M., Elliott, K.-E., Andrews, S., Stirling, C., Ashby, M., Donohue, C., Banks, S., Toye, C., and Mcinerney, F. (2014) 'Who knows, who cares? Dementia knowledge among nurses, care workers, and family members of people living with dementia', *Journal of Palliative Care*, 30: 158–65.

Scott, I., Cooper, C., Leverton, M., Burton, A., Beresford-Dent, J., Rockwood, K., Butler, L., and Rapaport, P. (2019) 'Effects of nonpharmacological interventions on functioning of people living with dementia at home: a systematic review of randomised controlled trials', *International Journal of Geriatric Psychiatry*, 34: 1386–402.

Shakespeare, T., Zeilig, H., and Mittler, P. (2017) 'Rights in mind: thinking differently about dementia and disability', *Dementia*, 18: 1075–88.

Smyth, W., Fielding, E., Beattie, E., Gardner, A., Moyle, W., Franklin, S., Hines, S., and Macandrew, M. (2013) 'A survey-based study of knowledge of Alzheimer's disease among health care staff', *BMC Geriatrics*, 13: 2.

Speechly, C.M., Bridges-Webb, C., and Passmore, E. (2008) 'The pathway to dementia diagnosis', *The Medical Journal of Australia*, 189: 487–9.

Szanton, S.L., Thorpe, R.J., Boyd, C., Tanner, E.K., Leff, B., Agree, E., Xue, Q.-L., Allen, J.K., Seplaki, C.L., Weiss, C.O., Guralnik, J.M., and Gitlin, L.N. (2011) 'Community aging in place, advancing better living for elders: a bio-behavioral-environmental intervention to improve function and health-related quality of life in disabled older adults', *Journal of the American Geriatrics Society*, 59: 2314–20.

Szanton, S.L., Wolff, J.W., Leff, B., Thorpe, R.J., Tanner, E.K., Boyd, C., Xue, Q., Guralnik, J., Bishai, D., and Gitlin, L.N. (2014) 'CAPABLE trial: a randomized controlled trial of nurse, occupational therapist and handyman to reduce disability among older adults: rationale and design', *Contemporary Clinical Trials*, 38: 102–12.

Taudorf, L., Nørgaard, A., Islamoska, S., Jørgensen, K., Laursen, T.M., and Waldemar, G. (2019) 'Declining incidence of dementia: a national registry-based study over 20 years', *Alzheimer's & Dementia*, 15: 1383–91.

Thuesen, J. (2021) 'Rehabilitering ved demens i let til moderat grad. Afrapportering af projektet DEM-REHAB' ['Rehabilitation in mild to moderate dementia. Report from the DEM-REHAB project'] [online], Available from: https://www.rehpa.dk/wp-content/uploads/2021/01/DEM-REHAB-slutrapport-FINAL.pdf.pdf.

Thuesen, J., Feiring, M., Doh, D., and Westendorp, R. (2021) 'Reablement in need of theories of ageing: would theories of successful ageing do?', *Journal of Ageing & Society*, 1–13. DOI: 10.1017/S0144686X21001203

United Nations (2006) *Convention on the Rights of Persons with Disabilities*, New York, NY: United Nations.

Van Hout, H.P., Vernooij-Dassen, M.J., and Stalman, W.A. (2007) 'Diagnosing dementia with confidence by GPs', *Family Practice*, 24: 616–21.

Vroomen, J.M., Bosmans, J.E., Van Hout, H.P.J., and De Rooij, S.E. (2013) 'Reviewing the definition of crisis in dementia care', *BMC Geriatrics*, 13: 10.

Warmoth, K., Morgan-Trimmer, S., Kudlicka, A., Toms, G., James, I.A., and Woods, B. (2020) 'Reflections on a personalized cognitive rehabilitation intervention: Experiences of people living with dementia and their carers participating in the GREAT trial', *Neuropsychological Rehabilitation*, 32(2): 268–84.

Werner, P. and Giveon, S.M. (2008) 'Discriminatory behavior of family physicians toward a person with Alzheimer's disease', *International Psychogeriatrics*, 20: 824–39.

World Health Organization (2012) *Dementia: A Public Health Priority*. Geneva, Switzerland: WHO [online], Available from: www.who.int.

World Health Organization (2017) *Global Action Plan on the Public Health Response to Dementia: 2017–2025*. Geneva, Switzerland: WHO [online], Available from: https://www.who.int/mental_health/neurology/dementia/action_plan_2017_2025/en/.

World Health Organisation (2020) *Dementia* [online]. Geneva, Switzerland: WHO [online], Available from: https://www.who.int/en/news-room/fact-sheets/detail/dementia.

Yang, L., Xuan, C., Yu, C., Jin, X., Zheng, P., and Yan, J. (2021) 'Effects of comprehensive intervention on life quality among the elderly with Alzheimer Disease and their caregivers based on mixed models', *Nursing Open*. DOI: 10.1002/nop2.917

9

Better care, better work?
Reablement in Danish home care and the implications for care workers

Tine Rostgaard and Lea Graff

Introduction

As covered elsewhere in the book, reablement has been introduced with the aim of improving functioning in daily activities for older people, and has implications for clients and their informal caregivers. However, it also has implications for formal care workers with respect to changing the aims and nature of their work, as well as introducing collaboration across different disciplines. The introduction of reablement could therefore potentially affect how attractive it is to work in the sector. This is highly relevant in an ageing world, where demographic changes are increasing the need for staff in the long-term care (LTC) sector as populations and the care workforce are ageing. There is currently a ratio of five LTC workers for every 100 people aged 65+ in the OECD countries, which extrapolates to an additional 13.5 million workers by 2040 (OECD, 2020). However, LTC work is generally characterised by insufficient staffing, poor working conditions, and low status and pay. The sector suffers from recruitment problems, high turnover, and subsequent staffing shortages, which will likely worsen soon. Attracting and retaining workers in the LTC sector is therefore a common concern in OECD countries (OECD, 2020), and reablement may be one solution to this.

This chapter primarily focuses on what the implications of the introduction of reablement are for home care workers, in the setting of Denmark where reablement has been implemented in home care since 2007. The chapter first investigates how reablement may affect care workers' approach to their work and what they consider to be good care, and the chapter thereafter considers the implications for how attractive they find the sector. Interview data from two municipalities and data from a national survey among care workers are applied. The results reveal how a common understanding has been established within the home care organisations: that furthering client self-reliance makes for more cost-effective interventions while also increasing their quality of life. Reablement appears to provide care workers with more professional autonomy and flexibility in the planning of their work while they also receive more support and attention from managers. The applied tasks and methods focus particularly on motivating the clients towards achieving such independence, and the reablement care workers find this both meaningful and professionally rewarding to the degree that they seem to be less likely to want to quit their job. The results are important, since there is otherwise a high turnover in the home care workforce, and it is difficult to recruit young people to the sector.

Setting the scene: long-term care and reablement care work in Denmark

LTC work in Denmark is mainly formal and organised according to the 'Public Service Model' principles, where the state (or rather, due to the extensive autonomy of local governments: the local municipality) is responsible for organising, financing, and largely also delivering care services (Anttonen, 1997). Overall, the Danish LTC system shares characteristics with other Nordic countries in offering service universalism whereby services such as home care are in principle attractive, affordable, and flexible (Vabø and Szebehely, 2012). Home care is therefore used across income and social class groupings (Rostgaard and Matthiessen, 2019). Denmark spends a relatively high proportion of Gross Domestic Product (GDP) on LTC (4.5 per cent of GDP), with 4 per cent of the 65+ population living in a nursing home and 11 per cent receiving home care. Home care consists of personal care (such as help with getting out of bed, bathing, getting dressed) and/ or practical assistance with household tasks, such as cleaning, laundry, and meal preparation.

In Denmark, reablement has been applied locally since 2007 and became part of the service act governing home care in 2015 (Social Services Act, section 83, 2014) (see also Chapters 2 and 3). Since then, municipalities must consider whether the older person has the so-called potential for reablement and, if not, regular home care is offered instead. The Danish application of reablement is in line with the Delphi definition of the term (Metzelthin et al, 2020; see also Chapter 1) and provides short-term and inter-disciplinary interventions, typically up to 12 weeks. The aim is to improve daily functioning based on the client's individual preferences and stated goals. As with regular home care, there is no charge for reablement services. In 2018, approximately 3 per cent of those aged 65+ received a reablement intervention, either as an alternative or supplement to home care. Alongside the introduction of reablement, overall coverage and hours for home care have been drastically reduced in recent years (Rostgaard and Matthiessen, 2019).

Reablement is usually provided by professional *home care workers*, who are also the central focus of this chapter. Home carers in Denmark are formally employed, and, relative to other countries, also reasonably well-paid and well-trained (Eurofound, 2020). Overall, 75 per cent of the LTC workforce have completed an education programme in social and healthcare. Of these, around half have 1.5 years of education as a 'social and healthcare helper' and another third are trained for 3.5 years as 'social and healthcare assistants'. The vast majority of home carers belong to one of these two professions. In Denmark, working in the LTC sector is considered to be a primary occupation and the vast majority of care staff are unionised (Dahl, 2009). Providing LTC for older people constitutes a substantial proportion of the Danish workforce, with more than 4 per cent of the workforce in 2017 working in this sector, and mainly women (Eurofound, 2020). In the reablement intervention, home carers work closely with physio- or occupational therapists and meet regularly.

Theoretical framework: from time-squeezed and standardised to more autonomous work

The Nordic care model is known for its generosity, however, as in other Nordic countries, the Danish LTC sector has been pressed to make services more cost-effective. New Public Management (NPM) steering principles have been applied since the 1980s to achieve this end, with emphasis on efficiency, documentation, and competitive tendering (Rostgaard et al, 2012; Hansen et al, 2021). Services have become more instrumental, with little time for relational care, which is often seen to be important for care rationality and therefore for the meaningfulness of care work (Wærness, 1984). The changes have also implied increasing standardisation across client groups and geographical territories. Standardisation processes may ensure more predictability, efficiency, accountability, and objectivity in the work (Timmermans and Epstein, 2010) and in this way may require less of the care worker in terms of the constant assessment of need and reflection over what the required intervention is. However, standardisation has also been criticised for creating a sense of mistrust regarding the quality and volume of the individual care worker's performance, and for taming their professional autonomy (Hvid and Kamp, 2012; Rostgaard, 2012). Taken together, these organisational changes seem to have affected the motivation for working in the sector, with increasing worker absence due to illness and problems recruiting and retaining staff as a result. For example, the 'social and health assistant' occupation is among the top five occupations with unfilled vacancies in Denmark (from among 576 occupations) (Eurofound, 2020), and a 2021 survey found that four times out of ten, municipalities were unable to hire personnel with the required competencies to work in the sector (Danish Agency for Labour Market and Recruitment, nd).

Reablement may constitute a game-changer, as it changes care work both in terms of how the work is organised, and in the aim, tasks, and methods required. Ideally, the aim of the reablement intervention is more holistic than regular home care and considers not only the client's physical needs but also cognitive and social needs, as these are also important for functional ability (Aspinal et al, 2016; Metzelthin et al, 2020). Compared to regular home care, the reablement approach focuses on a clear, measurable output; that is, an improvement in functional ability, which may motivate client and care worker alike. In so doing, reablement is in accordance with NPM guiding principles for setting up clear targets and goals for the work output and measuring ongoing progress as a means of steering and extrinsically motivating the employee (Bøgh-Andersen et al, 2017). In reablement, however, there are also elements that the NPM approach has valued less: there is a strong element of relational work, as the intervention requires a close relationship with the care clients to learn their preferences and motivation. In principle, as reablement work is less standardised, there may also be more professional autonomy in the planning and carrying out of the work. In this way, care provision could become more personalised and less bureaucratic. Moreover, as it is an interdisciplinary intervention, it involves close cooperation, communication, and learning opportunities from working in teams with peers and other professions (such as occupational- and physiotherapists). These elements may appeal to the use and upgrading of professional skills, as well as ensuring that care work becomes less automatised.

Such elements also speak directly to what Evetts (2011) generally describes as a new understanding of professionalism, where the ideologies of employee empowerment, autonomy, and discretion are dominant, as a means to achieve innovation and improve quality and customer care. Sitting well with Friedson's understanding of professionalism as a social organisation (Friedson, 2001), it is also an ideal understanding of professionalism where there is negotiation between complex numbers of professional agencies and interests. Rather than letting a mono-disciplinary ownership of professionalism constitute the social organisation of care work, ideally the professional ownership and advocacy of practice is shared across disciplines.

When translating Evetts' ideas to the case of reablement, the complexity lies is in the need to align goals and perspectives not only with the client and their family but also with other professions, such as occupational- and physiotherapists as well as with the overall goal of the organisation. However, across these agencies and interests, there is a commonly acknowledged aim: to support older people in becoming independent in their daily activities, a goal that can hardly be disputed. As Evetts describes, the new understanding of professionalism, therefore, implies that the interest of the organisation becomes closely intertwined with that of the professional. This can be seen in contrast to Abbott's (1988) classical description of *occupational* professionalism, where the protection of professional monopoly, status, and power meant that the interests of the organisation could well differ from those of the profession. In her account of new professionalism, Evetts (2011) argues that the new form of *organisational* professionalism instead ensures that the professional and organisational logics and values are more aligned. This also means that the control of professionals can be achieved by means of employee self-regulation and allowing employees to compete with themselves (and others) on individual performance (Evetts, 2011). Translating Evetts' ideas regarding organisational professionalism to the reablement case means that as organisational and individual interests are more aligned, the reablement organisation can resort to more intrinsic forms of care worker motivation. With this approach, there is general agreement across the organisation and between professionals that successful performance on behalf of the care worker results in the creation of more functional, able-bodied clients to the degree they require less home care and, in some cases, no services at all. A success for the individual care worker is eventually a success for the organisation. Facilitating such client self-reliance may therefore be a strong intrinsic motivation factor for the care worker.

Conversely, reablement requires fine-tuned interpersonal skills in the relationship with the client, especially when they are less motivated to participate in the intervention. The individual care worker is predominantly alone with the responsibility for co-producing client self-reliance, regardless of how much they are supported by their peers and other professions. This means that using the terminology from the governmentality literature, there is a process of 'responsibilisation' in care work (Rose, 2000). Reablement is also to be delivered in an organisational context still heavily influenced by the NPM emphasis on cost-effectiveness and time optimisation, and there may not always be enough time set aside for working with the client to help them improve functional independence. Also, as is well established in the literature, interdisciplinary work may blur professional boundaries (Nancarrow and Borthwick, 2005) and create role conflicts that lead to stress and job dissatisfaction (Carpenter et al, 2012). In the reablement case, interdisciplinary work may therefore weaken the already less strong professional identity of the home carers and add to their levels of stress and hurt their job satisfaction. The reablement approach may therefore positively or negatively impact the attractiveness of care work and the recruitment and retention of care workers in a work sector also struggling with ageing and early retirement due to increasing demands and burnout. From an employee perspective, this chapter, therefore, aims first to understand what reablement entails regarding understandings of good care and the professional tasks and methods involved, and second, to consider the implications for whether reablement care workers view their work as attractive with respect to meeting individual client needs, receiving support from managers, and for their intentions to continue to work in the sector.

Methodology

To answer this, quantitative and qualitative data are used. The qualitative study was conducted as ethnographic case studies in the home care sector in two Danish municipalities in 2015–2016. The aim was to investigate what the introduction of reablement meant for work practices. The two municipalities were strategically chosen based on their reablement efforts being well-established, well-functioning, as well as having a strong focus on interdisciplinary reablement work. In this way, what Flyvbjerg (2006) calls paradigmatic cases are applied, which allows the making of generalised statements. The study builds on literature studies, 13 focus and 28 individual interviews with clients and professionals, and 13 observational studies of interdisciplinary reablement meetings (see also Rostgaard and Graff, 2016).

This chapter primarily draws on seven individual and five group interviews with, in total, 18 care workers working in the home care sector (one male, 17 female). The care workers all had prior experience with working in regular home care services as well and were primarily trained as social and health helpers (12) and social and healthcare assistants (5). In addition to training in reablement as part of their formal education, they had received additional on-the-job training (6 days in one municipality, 11 days in the other). The care workers were recruited to the study by the municipalities based on their experience with reablement work. Two group interviews with top-level and middle-level managers were also carried out. The interviews were all coded and thematically analysed. The study followed Danish research guidelines for qualitative studies and the Danish Data Protection Agency regulations.

For the quantitative approach, the Danish data from a representative survey conducted in 2015 as part of the Nordic NORDCARE study are applied. The data were collected by postal questionnaire, which was sent to a randomised sample of unionised care workers working in the LTC sector. The sample came from membership registers of the care union, Forbundet af Offentligt Ansatte (FOA) (nurses, physiotherapists, and occupational therapists were not part of the sample, as they belong to different unions). Care workers working in the private for-profit sector were underrepresented in the sample. The Danish sample size was 1,130 persons working in home care and nursing homes (59.3 per cent response rate). This chapter only applies the home care worker data (361). The survey questions generally focused on care work tasks, quality of care, and intentions to continue working in the care sector. Since municipalities organise reablement in numerous ways, the analysis does not compare care workers in regular home care with care workers working with reablement. Instead, the analysis examines how often care workers in general applied the reablement approach in their work, according to the survey question 'How often do you motivate a client to participate in a reablement/help-to-self-help intervention?'. In the survey, 27.3 per cent reported that they provided such assistance several times a day, 48.8 per cent provided it every day, 12.1 per cent every week, 5.4 per cent every month, and 6.4 per cent less often. Care workers who often provided reablement were more often employed in the public sector, while there was no significant difference in educational background. The analysis compares the frequency of providing reablement with a number of items, including the meaningfulness of work and retention intentions. The logistic regression analysis controls for differences in work hours and private for-profit versus public employment, age, gender, work experience, and education.

One limitation of the study is that the qualitative interviews are restricted to only home care workers working with reablement. It is possible that these individuals were recruited (for their jobs and the interviews alike) by the municipalities because they were strong proponents of this particular approach, which may create a selection bias in the accounts of working with reablement. As mentioned previously, however, the presentation of the survey data also includes those home care workers with little or no experience with reablement.

We first report the findings from the qualitative interviews to illustrate how the introduction of reablement has advanced new understandings of care needs, new tasks, and the application of new professional skills and methods before applying the quantitative data to investigate the implications for whether care workers view care work as attractive.

Results from the qualitative study

New and common understandings of care needs and how to meet them

It became apparent in the care worker interviews that the introduction of reablement in Danish home care has promoted new understandings of care needs and how these needs are best met. In contrast with former care practices focusing on performing care tasks *for* instead of *with* the care recipient, the care workers who work with reablement were now continuously oriented towards the optimisation of care clients' functional abilities and generally considered reablement an efficient approach to support self-reliance in older people. When reflecting on the benefits of reablement, they primarily referred to increased quality of life, presenting this primarily as being independent of care and able to make autonomous decisions for oneself or, as one care worker said: 'once again being master of the house'. The care workers expressed their appreciation of how reablement had (re-)introduced a more holistic and individualised approach to care, which they found more attentive to a wider range of individual needs and preferences than usual practice:

> 'The softer values are also in focus now; those things that weren't measurable – quality of life. We can support people in getting out of the house again or that they can begin to cook their own meals. Or, if they enjoyed putting on nail polish, maybe we can support that so they can begin to do it again.' (Care worker A, municipality X)

New forms of relationships

A new awareness of the individual clients and their life situation, as in the quote from care worker A, is linked to the relationship between care workers and clients. Since the intervention is primarily carried out by the same person, the care workers felt they had a better understanding of the client's preferences and their motivational 'triggers'. As one care worker explained, 'I don't think I had this kind of relationship with the clients before. You just went in, did your work, and then left again' (care worker B, municipality X). The closer relationship also enables an awareness about the need to break old habits, also among care staff themselves. One care worker described how, before the introduction of reablement, she would often just stick to her given list of tasks, such as serving one care client porridge for breakfast (as she had done for years), until one day she started wondering whether that was actually the client's preferred choice:

> 'I accidentally asked her … [and she said] "Um, I'd actually like to have two cheese sandwiches and a cup of coffee. You're the first to ever ask me". … It was a bit of shock for me. After that, I started asking people what they would like for breakfast.' (Care worker C, municipality X)

According to the care workers, they often found that they developed close relationships with the clients despite the short timeframe for the interventions. This meant that they could individualise the interventions, and it opened their eyes to care for clients' preferences in general.

Facilitating change as a meaningful practice

Supporting change in the daily lives of those to whom care is provided and seeing development as the intervention progressed were mentioned as two of the most satisfying elements of reablement work. Facilitating change – instead of compensating for decline – made the work more meaningful for the care workers. In fact, the workers agreed on reablement being beneficial not only to the clients but to themselves as well. Supporting people in regaining their independence and seeing their quality of life improve was professionally satisfying. This was also beneficial for the care workers' professional self-esteem, as illustrated in the following excerpt from an interview with three municipality X care workers:

Care worker D: I think this is a great way to work.
Care worker E: This is the right way to do it.
Interviewer: For you and the citizens both?
Care worker D: For both parties. You know, it damn well adds to your self-esteem when you follow a client throughout the intervention, you can let them go, and they can manage on their own … It gives so much to both parties. After all, they're also really happy to be able to take care of themselves again after the intervention.

Introduction of new tasks and methods

Reablement has not only affected perceptions of care needs and how these should be met; it has also had a profound impact on the content of care staff work and has necessitated the development of new motivational methods when working with the clients. A client being motivated to become as self-reliant as possible is often presented as a prerequisite for a successful intervention (Rabiee and Glendinning, 2011; Newton, 2012; Tuntland et al, 2016; Hjelle et al, 2017; Stausholm et al, 2021). This means that a new task for care staff is motivating clients to participate in the intervention. At the time of the study, it seemed that these motivational methods had yet to develop fully, and care workers had to rely somewhat instead on coming up with their own.

It became apparent in the interviews that the care workers had embraced the importance of client motivation. To motivate clients, they drew on multiple methods, often based on trial and error from their daily practice and often based on personal (rather than professional) skills. The main new method for getting people to perform certain activities (such as bathing or preparing food themselves) was the 'hands in the pockets-approach', a wait-and-see tactic contrasting former care approaches, where tasks were, it was argued, performed for the client before they had even articulated a need. Other ways to motivate clients included deliberately delaying visits or 'forgetting' to perform a task, thereby challenging perceived client dependence on assistance to perform the given task, possibly making them perform it unassisted. This would allow the care worker to point out and praise the client for being able to perform the activity themselves. Working in reablement necessitated coming up with and applying a range of new and innovative methods, which care workers described as satisfying:

> 'You continuously have to think outside the box. Think about new ideas and approaches. Think about what to do if this doesn't work – can we do something else? Small things can make a difference, and that's what you need to keep thinking about here.' (Care worker F, municipality X)

The introduction of reablement thus meant new and more challenging tasks and fewer standardised routine tasks for the care workers.

Cooperation with therapists

The implementation of reablement also entailed new and close cooperation across professions. The care workers particularly highlighted the close cooperation with occupational therapists and physiotherapists, which they described as a major factor in the successful implementation of reablement. The cooperation with therapists also added to their professional skillset; they drew on the therapists' advice and expertise in assessing needs and relevant approaches:

> 'It [working with reablement] gets easier and easier, because you learn from how they see things. I can give an example: a client had difficulties sitting down on the toilet, because she felt it was very low. And then you immediately think: "Well, maybe she needs a toilet aid that raises it". But seeing it from the therapist's perspective: that might not be good, because you use your muscles sitting down and getting up again. That's obviously all related to training. And that makes us care workers better at thinking about training in each intervention.' (Care worker G, municipality Y)

The increased interdisciplinary collaboration, therefore, did not from the interviews seem to cause any job dissatisfaction or create role conflicts. Instead, the care workers largely appeared to adopt the professional language and approach of their therapist colleagues.

The managers did not generally find that the adoption of the therapists' approaches posed any risks of blurring the care workers professional boundaries. Instead, they emphasised the ability of the care workers to work across disciplines and how this actually required strong mono–disciplinary skills, which they found the care workers possessed fully. According to managers and care workers alike, the therapists likewise appreciated the care worker professionalism and their knowledge of each client, and they would draw on their assistance and advice on how to support a given client's progress.

Managerial support

The new roles for care workers as motivators and front-line 'enforcers' of the reablement policy, also towards potentially critical clients and relatives, strengthens the need for managerial support, a topic emphasised by managers in both municipalities. They put considerable effort into supporting reablement care staff, who often had to convince clients, relatives, and colleagues in the regular home care services that reablement was the right approach to achieve functional independence.

> 'It takes a lot of support for the care workers, especially when they have to have those conversations. Because they really have to be prepared and supported in arguing 'That's right, and you have to do and …'. Because sometimes they find it hard to place demands on the clients. But in this case, it's actually a *demand* to the client – "this is how we do it".' (Manager A, municipality Y)

A top-level manager likewise emphasised that the care workers should always rest assured that they had full managerial support: 'When you go out and ask the clients to perform the tasks themselves, then we are fully behind you' (manager B, municipality X). In both municipalities, managers focused on continuously supporting care workers, such as by training them to be advocates for the benefits of reablement or in how to articulate the demands to clients. Besides training and day-to-day support, managers also offered support via reablement meetings. The introduction of reablement entailed an increase in meetings due to the heightened need for mono- and interdisciplinary coordination. Since managers were present in these meetings, care workers had more access to professional support from them than usual.

Prestige of reablement work

In the literature, reablement work is often highlighted for offering care workers new and strengthened professional identities with higher status compared to ordinary home care work (Hansen, 2016; Hansen and Kamp, 2016; Jensen and Muhr, 2020). Higher status stems from working close to the therapists' professional expertise, which lends the care workers new techniques and more challenging tasks (Hansen and Kamp, 2016; Jensen and Muhr, 2020) as well as from reablement care work's distance to traditionally stigmatised physical care work (Hansen, 2016; Jensen, 2017). Organisationally, the two case municipalities have aimed to heighten the prestige of working with reablement in order to attract competent care workers, as well as to underline the 'shift' in care culture. For instance, one of the municipalities introduced specially coloured uniforms for the reablement teams so that they stood out, publicly celebrated when staff finalised a reablement training course, and generally highlighted reablement in policy papers where possible. In the interviews, care workers emphasised how working with reablement was attractive for them since it was a work position, which to a larger degree gained recognition from middle-management and which, in their experience, was increasingly valued by colleagues in other home care departments as well. However, the organisational practices underlining the differences in status could, in the interviewed care workers' experience, initially add to the mistrust and uncertainty from regular home care workers being nervous about whether the new approach posed a risk to their job security. But they also experienced that the distance and differences seemed to diminish over time as the reablement mindset spread across the home care organisation.

Professional autonomy and flexibility

Another factor highlighted by the care workers as influencing their overall positive attitude towards reablement work, was the differences in professional autonomy in reablement versus in regular home care. Studies from New Zealand (King et al, 2012) and Norway (Vik, 2018) have highlighted how care workers experienced increased job satisfaction due to the higher degree of flexibility and autonomy in their daily work. These findings were mirrored in this study. Often, care workers would point out that working with reablement led to higher degrees of professional autonomy and influence on their workday – especially as they did not have the same time constraints as their colleagues working with regular home care, where each part of the service was allotted a fixed time-slot, for example, 12 minutes for helping with lunch: 'Since we don't operate with fixed time-slots, we add the services we assess to be necessary ourselves. We add or remove time for the services ourselves based on what is needed' (care worker D, municipality X).

The autonomy thus also made for more flexible interventions: 'In general, it generates more flexibility – also in terms of planning – that there's enough time. And we arrange things between ourselves if we experience delays' (care worker E, municipality X). That reablement care staff could not only dispose over their own time but also assess the need for services themselves, points towards a high degree of organisational trust in them. This trust also extended to allowing the care workers to assess and report back whether the service delivery should be adjusted.

Summarising, the qualitative study shows that a new, common understanding of care needs and approaches has been established in the two home care organisations. The interviewed care workers highlighted how the introduction of reablement enabled them to apply more flexibility and professional autonomy, backed up by their therapist colleagues and managers. They gained self-esteem from working with reablement and generally working as change facilitators.

Results from the survey study: implications of working with reablement for attractiveness of care work

This begs the question whether the introduction of reablement also has implications for how care workers view work in the sector as being attractive or not. To investigate this, the following sections apply the quantitative data from the national survey conducted among a representative sample of unionised home care workers, with varying degrees of experience working with reablement.

Meaningfulness in care work

This allows for the determination of whether the reablement approach (among others) contributes to the overall meaningfulness of LTC work. Figure 9.1 illustrates the clear association between how often home care workers provide reablement and how interesting and meaningful they find the work. For instance, among the care workers providing reablement several times daily, 83 per cent found their job interesting and meaningful, compared to only 57 per cent among those who provide reablement 'less often or never'. As seen from the qualitative interviews, this may be related to having flexibility in facilitating change and development among clients, and also being able to draw on the interdisciplinary collaboration with other peers and professions. The transparency and organisational alignment in what the desired output is, that is facilitating client self-reliance, may also contribute to the sense of meaningfulness, as may the greater autonomy in the planning of work, as described in the qualitative interviews.

Meeting client needs

Another explanation for why those working with reablement find that application of reablement makes their work more interesting and meaningful seems to be because they also find that the approach enables them to meet client needs in a better way, as the findings in Figures 9.2 and 9.3 suggest.

Figure 9.2 illustrates whether respondents found that the changes in opportunities to meet client needs had worsened or improved in recent

Figure 9.1: Finding work interesting and meaningful, relative to the frequency of providing reablement. Home care workers, per cent

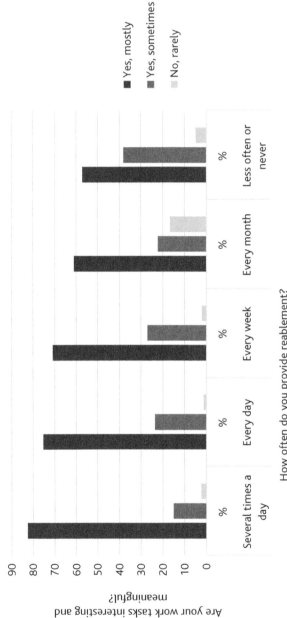

Note: Based on a logistic regression analysis. Significant on a 5 per cent level for home care workers who 'several times a day' and 'every day' provide reablement compared to all other home care workers. *n* = 338.

Figure 9.2: Changes in opportunities for meeting client needs in recent years, relative to the frequency of providing reablement. Home care workers, per cent

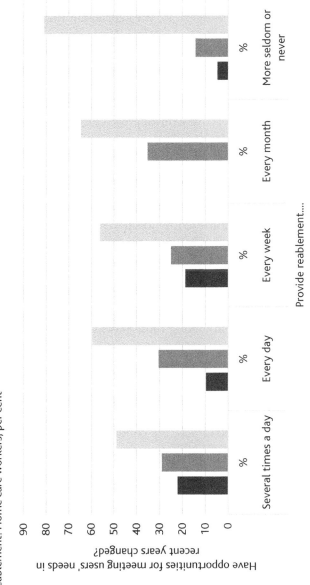

Note: Based on a logistic regression analysis. Significant on a 5 per cent level for home care workers who 'several times a day' provide reablement, compared to all other home care workers, for the response category 'overall improved' and 'overall worsened'. *n* = 336.

years. Overall, there is clearly a general – and worrying – feeling among home care workers that the conditions for meeting client needs have deteriorated over time. However, when crossing this with how often they provide reablement, there was a small but significant relationship between the two items, where those who provide reablement 'several times a day' stands out. Among these care workers, 22 per cent found that they could better meet client needs today; in contrast only 5 per cent of those who provided reablement 'monthly or more seldom' felt they could fulfil the client's needs. Likewise, among those who found that they were less able over time to meet the client's needs, fewer provided reablement on a regular basis. As reablement involves providing care according to the client's goals and preferences, the care workers using this approach seem to find that they can better meet the client's needs.

Providing individualised care

Figure 9.3 supports the argument that the ability to meet client needs is more closely related to the more personalised approach in reablement. The figure presents the care worker assessments of whether they are able to provide care according to individual needs. Here again, there is a close relationship between the frequency of which they provide reablement and whether they found that they provide for individual needs. Of those providing reablement every day, 41 per cent agreed that they provided individualised care, whereas this figure was only 19 per cent among those providing reablement on a monthly basis.

These results indicate that the involvement of the clients in stating their preferences and goals contributed to the understanding among care workers that individual needs were being met. As in the example provided in the qualitative section of the reablement care worker remembering to ask the client what her preferred breakfast was, the continuous attention to client individuality represents a cultural shift that the care workers providing reablement may find enriching.

Meetings with manager

Other organisational factors can also contribute to whether a job is attractive, including managerial attention. The qualitative interviews revealed how there was more managerial focus on the care workers providing reablement, both in terms of heightening the status of the work and in terms of offering support to the care workers. Due to an increase in team meetings stemming from the need for mono- as well as interdisciplinary collaboration on the reablement interventions, reablement care workers had more meetings with their managers. And the survey results seem to support this finding. Figure 9.4

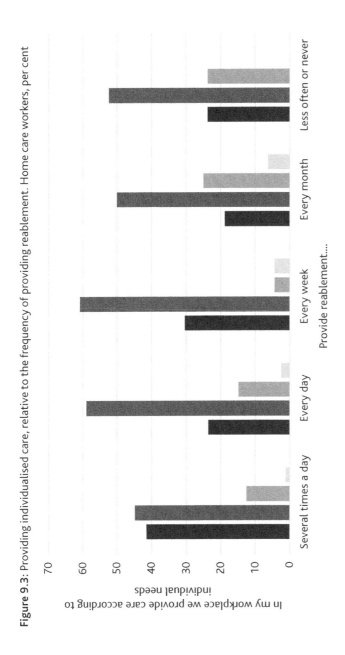

Figure 9.3: Providing individualised care, relative to the frequency of providing reablement. Home care workers, per cent

Note: Based on a logistic regression analysis. Significant on a 5 per cent level for home care workers who 'several times a day' and 'every day' provide reablement compared to all other home care workers. *n* = 331.

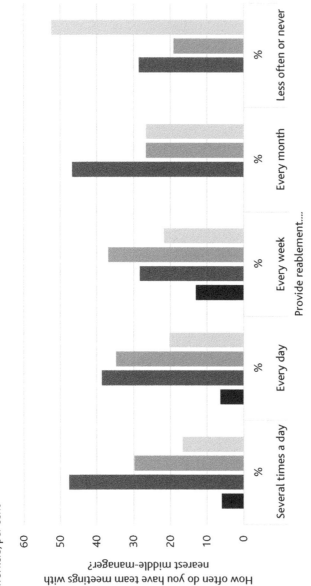

Figure 9.4: Have team meeting with middle manager, relative to the frequency of providing reablement. Home care workers, per cent

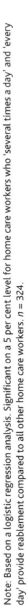

Note: Based on a logistic regression analysis. Significant on a 5 per cent level for home care workers who 'several times a day' and 'every day' provide reablement compared to all other home care workers. *n* = 324.

shows that care workers who more frequently provided reablement were also more likely to have team meetings with their middle manager. For example, 54 per cent of those who provided reablement on a daily basis also met with their manager daily or at minimum weekly, while this was only the case for 29 per cent of those rarely providing reablement.

Receiving support from manager

The care workers who were more frequently involved in reablement also found more often that they received support from their middle manager. The interviews revealed a strong focus among the managers on continuously supporting the care workers, both in day-to-day practice and in reablement meetings. Figure 9.5 shows that only 18 per cent of those who worked with reablement every day indicated that they rarely or never received managerial support, compared to 41 per cent of those who rarely provided reablement. As the qualitative interviews revealed, one indication of such support was also that care workers were trusted within the organisation to determine their time and plan how their work should be carried out, in stark contrast to regular home carers.

Intentions to quit job

Finally, there was a clear relationship between how often a care worker provided reablement and whether they seriously considered quitting their job. Indicative of the generally poor working conditions in the home care sector, a relatively large percentage of home care workers indicated in the survey that they were considering leaving their job, 43 per cent in total. As Figure 9.6 shows, however, this was significantly lower among those more frequently providing reablement. In the regression analysis, higher age and problems with work–family life balance were also significant for wanting to quit.

Taking into consideration the previous analyses, this indicates that the meaningfulness of providing reablement, the ability to better meet individual needs, and the general support and focus from managers, may contribute to workplace retention in this sector. It may eventually also improve sector recruitment.

All in all, the quantitative data seem to support the qualitative findings in that care workers have a generally positive assessment of working with reablement. Care workers providing reablement on a frequent basis are highly likely to find their work attractive with respect to meeting individual client needs, receiving support from managers, and for their sense of meaningfulness and the intention to continue in the sector.

Figure 9.5: Support from middle manager, relative to the frequency of providing reablement. Home care workers, per cent

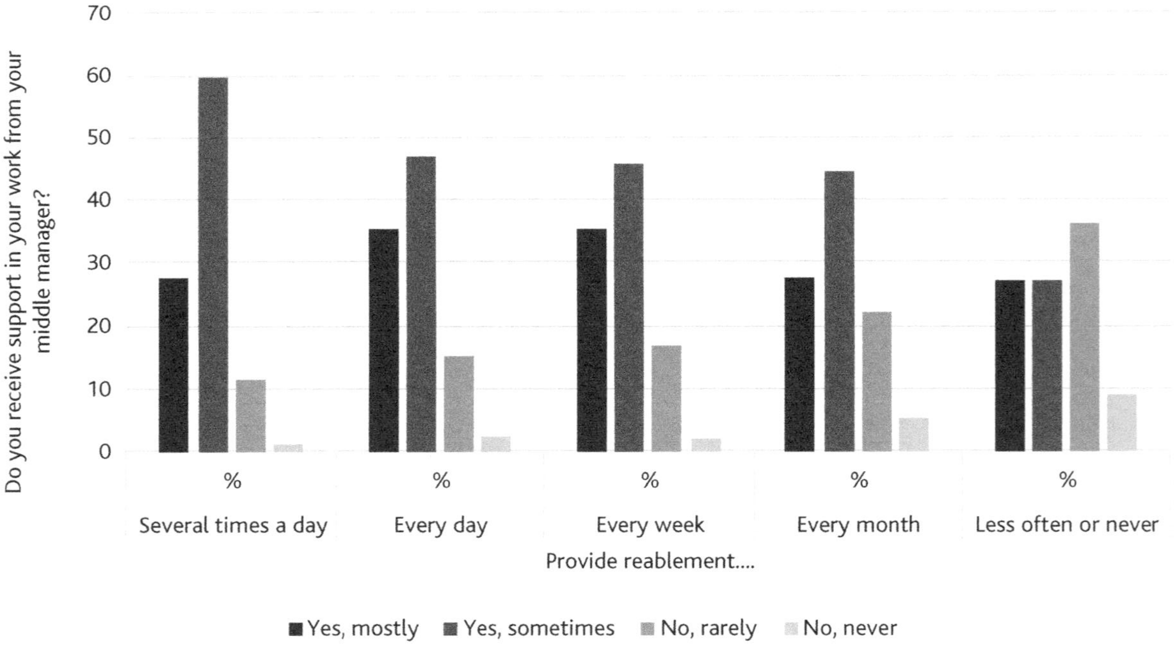

Note: Based on a logistic regression analysis. Significant on a 5 per cent level for home care workers who 'several times a day' and 'every day' provide reablement compared to all other home care workers with respect to receiving support ('yes, most of the time' and 'yes, some times') and not receiving support ('no, rarely' and 'no, never'. n = 339.

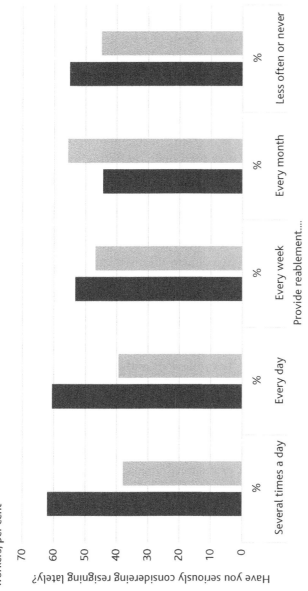

Figure 9.6: Have lately seriously considered resigning, relative to the frequency of providing reablement. Home care workers, per cent

Note: Based on a logistic regression analysis. Significant on a 5 per cent level for home care workers who 'several times a day' and 'every day' provide reablement compared to all other home care workers. *n* = 337.

Discussion

There is a need for more care workers in the LTC sector, in Denmark and the other OECD countries. The data shown in this chapter indicate that implementing reablement could lead to improvements in the retention and recruitment of care workers to the sector. There are numerous reasons for this: reablement changes the focus of care provision in a way that professional and organisational aims are better aligned. In accordance with Evetts' (2011) argument, the creation of such new organisational professionalism ensures that the individual professional and organisation apply similar logics and values and have matching means to an end. In particular, the care workers highlight the intention of adding to the client's quality of life, rather than seeing the facilitation of independence in daily tasks as mainly an organisational cost-saving manoeuvre. Very importantly, this means that there is a shared criterion of success and that the reablement organisation has less need to apply the traditional NPM extrinsic forms to motivate care workers. The qualitative data showed that successfully acting as a change facilitator and ensuring that clients become more self-reliant is a central part of how these care workers approach their work and seem to add to their self-esteem and satisfaction with their work.

New methods were developed and applied, particularly methods in how to motivate clients to better understand and manage their daily tasks on their own. And despite standing relatively alone with developing such new methods, care workers generally appreciated the reablement approach and felt comfortable in their new role. Part of the new confidence among care workers seemed to stem from the working relationship with the therapists, which gave the care workers new professional tools and support to 'think outside the box'. The increased interdisciplinary collaboration does not seem to cause job dissatisfaction (on the contrary), but it may not have contributed to strengthening professional boundaries, as care workers seemed to adopt the professional language and approach from their therapist colleagues rather than developing their own. Their professional boundaries may therefore have become somewhat blurred (Nancarrow and Borthwick, 2005). Regardless, care workers seem to have gained recognition, not only as the 'daily life experts', as their therapist colleagues called them; they were also singled out positively in the organisation in a different way than their colleagues who provide regular care. And very importantly, they seemed to have more flexibility in the organisation of their work and to be able to apply more professional autonomy as to when and how their work is carried out, mirroring Evetts' understanding of new professionalism where employee empowerment, autonomy, and discretion are dominant values; this in contrast to the normal practice in the otherwise NPM-ridden home care sector and its focus on cost-effectiveness and time optimisation.

As the survey data established, there was a clear relationship between the frequency of providing reablement and finding the work meaningful. Explanations for this seem to include the ability to meet the client's needs and providing more individualised care. Working with reablement also adds to the likelihood of being 'seen' and recognised by management, as these workers met more often with their middle manager and therefore received more support than their colleagues delivering more conventional home care. And not least, those working frequently with reablement were less likely to want to quit their job. These findings are in line with other studies of reablement and work conditions, such as those from New Zealand (King et al, 2012), where care workers in a restorative home care intervention were found to have reduced turnover rates and improved job satisfaction due to, among other factors, a higher degree of flexibility. Norway offers another example, where Vik (2018), in a study of interdisciplinary reablement work, found that a higher degree of flexibility and autonomy improves the working conditions and care worker commitment.

However, despite all the benefits that the care workers experienced from the implementation of reablement, the study in hand also indicates certain potentially critical organisational issues, such as a lack of opportunity for the development of own professional skills, 'responsibilisation' for client outcomes, and the risk of dichotomisation and devaluing of regular home care practices.

Although the care workers interviewed generally appreciated the more challenging tasks associated with reablement, their application of methods to motivate clients also occasionally appeared slightly arbitrary. Although trained care workers in Denmark have received extensive formal education, they have often received little or no training in reablement during their education or in the workplace, which apparently did not suffice in terms of allowing them to acquire shared professional skills for motivational work. In practice, they often came up with their own situational solutions based on personal (rather than professional) skills. Even though organisational measures (such as interdisciplinary reablement meetings) to ensure collaboration were present, the care workers usually worked alone. Thus, they had to make the situational decisions on motivational methods on their own, balancing between respecting the older person's integrity while continuously pushing them towards the goal of progress. The interviews and observations of reablement practice produced examples (some mentioned previously) of motivational methods bordering on the unethical, such as deliberately delaying visits and then not being upfront with the client about the real reason, or other somewhat infantilising approaches to the clients (such as praising them extensively, as one would a child). Should something go wrong (such as a client is injured trying to perform a 'delayed' or 'forgotten' task themselves), the responsibility is on the individual care worker instead of the organisation for not providing sufficient support and training for the development of professional skills.

Another challenge was that the assessment of the care workers' individual performance was tied to successful client outcomes. This has implications for how different clients are perceived. As studies have pointed out (Rabiee and Glendinning, 2011; Tuntland et al, 2016; Stausholm et al, 2021), reablement seems most beneficial for those who are highly motivated to regain their full independence. People less motivated are far more challenging to 'reable', and some care workers actually referred to this group as 'heavy clients' and as being less satisfying to work with. The emphasis on reducing dependency among clients also affects work performance assessments. If the individual performance of care workers is assessed according to their ability to motivate clients to work towards self-reliance, lack of motivation on behalf of the client might be viewed as a poor result of the care worker's approach instead of considering whether reablement was the right intervention for this client to begin with.

Reablement organisations might also want to pay attention to whether they inadvertently contribute to the dichotomisation between the valorised reablement approach and the oft-criticised regular home care approaches. Danish studies of the introduction of reablement have highlighted how managerial discourses and healthcare professionals position reablement work as a desirable and 'good' care practice compared to ordinary home care work, which is positioned as a 'bad' care practice that may 'pacify' clients (Jensen, 2017; Bødker et al, 2019). These studies also argue that the normative positioning of reablement as superior to ordinary home care work risks reinforcing both the stigma related to care work (Jensen, 2017; Bødker et al, 2019) as well as the perception of ordinary home care work as 'less professional' (Hansen and Kamp, 2016; Jensen and Muhr, 2020) and call for more nuanced views recognising the complementarity and necessity of both care approaches (Hansen and Kamp, 2016; Bødker et al, 2019). These discourses were also found in this study. In the interviews, care workers heavily emphasised never wanting to return to working with regular home care approaches. This was obviously due to how they liked working with reablement, but the benefits of reablement were often presented in terms of the contrast with regular home care approaches. The interviewed managers did attempt to soften the division by emphasising the need for both approaches depending on the client needs. As the survey data showed, however, in terms of the frequency of meeting up with managers, the organisation focused more on those care workers providing reablement, which implies easier access to managerial attention.

Conclusion

Other chapters in the book have found that the application of reablement may provide better care for clients (see Chapter 5 by Lewin et al and Chapter 7 by Zingmark et al), as the approach is more personalised and goal-oriented. This study suggests that reablement may also provide a path forward towards addressing the substantive and global problem of shortage of care workers in the LTC sector. As the study identified, however, there are new risks associated with reablement work. The professionals stand more alone in producing the desired output (such as increasing client independence in daily tasks), even for those clients who are less inclined to be 'reabled'. At times, it is with the means of inventive but nevertheless self-made motivational experiments based more on personal than professional skills. The study, therefore, suggests the need for continuous organisational focus on developing professional skills in reablement. It also suggests the need to acknowledge that reablement work can be successful also when it does not lead to less dependency but 'just' better quality of life for the client. In this way, better care for the client may imply better work for the care worker – also in the future. For care organisations struggling to recruit and retain staff (and regardless of whether they apply the full approach of reablement), the lessons produced here are that stronger professional autonomy and the application of a goal-oriented, person-centred approach are elements that may pave the way.

References

Abbott, A. (1988) *The System of Professions: An Essay on the Division of Expert Labor*, Chicago: University of Chicago Press.

Anttonen, A. (1997) 'The welfare state and social citizenship', in K. Kauppinen and T. Gordon (eds) *Unresolved Dilemmas: Women, Work and the Family in the United States, Europe and the Former Soviet Union*, Aldershot: Ashgate, pp 9–32.

Aspinal, F., Glasby, J., Rostgaard, T., Tuntland, H., and Westendorp, R. (2016) 'New horizons: reablement – supporting older people towards independence', *Age and Ageing*, 45(5): 574-8.

Bødker, M.N., Langstrup, H., and Christensen, U. (2019) 'What constitutes "good care" and "good carers"? The normative implications of introducing reablement in Danish home care', *Health & Social Care in the Community*, 27: e871-8. DOI: 10.1111/hsc.12815

Bøgh-Andersen, L., Torfing, J., Klaudi, K., and Greve, C. (2017) *Offentlige styringsparadigmer: Konkurrence og sameksistens*, Copenhagen: Djøf Publishing.

Carpenter, J., Webb, C., and Bostock, L. (2012) '*Effective Supervision in Social Work and Social Care*', London: Social Care Institute for Excellence, Research Briefing 43.

Dahl, H.M. (2009) 'New Public Management, care and struggles about recognition', *Critical Social Policy*, 29(4): 634–54.

Danish Agency for Labour Market and Recruitment (nd) 'Succesfulde og forgæves rekrutteringer' [online], Available from: https://star.dk/viden-og-tal/udvikling-paa-arbejdsmarkedet/rekrutteringssurveys/

Eurofound (2020) '*Long-term Care Workforce: Employment and Working Conditions*', Luxembourg: Publications Office of the European Union.

Evetts, J. (2011) 'A new professionalism? Challenges and opportunities', *Current Sociology*, 59(4): 406–22.

Flyvbjerg, B. (2006) 'Five misunderstandings about case-study research', in *Qualitative Inquiry*, 12(2): 219–45.

Friedson, E. (2001) '*Professionalism: The Third Logic*', Chicago: University of Chicago Press.

Hansen, A.M. (2016) 'Rehabilitative bodywork: cleaning up the dirty work of homecare', *Sociology of Health & Illness*, 38(7): 1092–105. DOI:10.1111/1467-9566.12435

Hansen, A.M. and Kamp, A. (2016) 'From carers to trainers: professional identity and body work in rehabilitative eldercare', *Gender, Work & Organization*. DOI:10.1111/gwao.12126

Hansen, L.L., Dahl, H.M., and Horn, L. (2021) *A Care Crisis in the Nordic Welfare States? Care Work, Gender Equality and Welfare State Sustainability*. Bristol: Policy Press.

Hjelle, K.M., Tuntland, H., Førland, O., and Avlsvåg, H. (2017) 'Driving forces for home-based reablement: a qualitative study of older adults' experiences', *Health & Social Care in the Community*, 25(5): 1581–9.

Hvid, H. and Kamp, A. (eds) (2012) *Elderly Care in Transition–Management, Meaning and Identity at Work. A Scandinavian Perspective*, Frederiksberg: Copenhagen Business School Press.

Jensen, M.C.F. (2017) 'Gender stereotypes and the reshaping of stigma in rehabilitative eldercare', *Gender, Work and Organization*, 24(6). DOI: 10.1111/gwao.12191

Jensen, M.C.F. and Muhr, S.L. (2020) 'Performative identity regulation in rehabilitative home care work: an analysis of how experts' embodied mediation of the managerial ideology "activates" new frontline identities', *Culture and Organization*, 26(3): 211–30.

King, A.I., Parsons, M., and Robinson, E. (2012) 'A restorative home care intervention in New Zealand: perceptions of paid caregivers', *Health & Social Care in the Community*, 20(1): 70–9.

Metzelthin, S., Rostgaard, T., Parsons, M., & Burton, E. (2020). 'Development of an internationally accepted definition of reablement: A Delphi study', *Ageing and Society*, 42(3): 703–18.

Nancarrow, S.A. and Borthwick, A.M. (2005) 'Dynamic professional boundaries in the healthcare workforce', *Sociology of Health & Illness*, 27(7): 897–919.

Newton, C. (2012) 'Personalising reablement: inserting the missing link', *Working with Older People*, 16(3): 117–21.

OECD (2020) *Who Cares? Attracting and Retaining Care Workers for the Elderly*, Paris: OECD.

Rabiee, P. and Glendinning, C. (2011) 'Organisation and delivery of home care re-ablement: what makes a difference?', *Health & Social Care in the Community*, 19(5): 495–503.

Rose, N. (2000) 'Government and control', *The British Journal of Criminology*, 40(2): 321–39.

Rostgaard, T. (2012) 'Quality reforms in Danish home care: balancing between standardisation and individualization', *Health & Social Care in the Community*, 20(3): 247–54.

Rostgaard, T. and Graff, L. (2016) *Med hænderne i lommen. Borger og medarbejders samspil og samarbejde i rehabilitering. Fremfærd rapport*. Copenhagen: VIVE [online], Available from: https://www.vive.dk/da/udgivelser/med-haende rne-i-lommen-8841/

Rostgaard, T. and Matthiessen, M. (2019) *Hjælp til svage ældre*. VIVE report. Copenhagen: VIVE.

Rostgaard, T., Timonen, V., and Glendinning, C. (2012) 'Guest editorial: reforming home care in ageing societies', *Health & Social Care in the Community*, 20(3): 225–7.

Social Services Act (2014) *Lov om ændring af lov om social service. Indenrigsministeriet. Lov nr 1524 af 27/12/2014*. Copenhagen: Retsinformation.

Stausholm, M.N., Pape-Haugaard, L., Hejlesen, O.K., and Heyckendorff Secher, P. (2021) 'Reablement professionals' perspectives on client characteristics and factors associated with successful home-based reablement: a qualitative study', *BMC Health Services Research*, 21: 665.

Timmermans, S. and Epstein, S. (2010) 'A world of standards but not a standard world: toward a sociology of standards and standardization', *Annual Review of Sociology*, 36(1): 69–89.

Tuntland, H., Kjeken, I., Langeland, E., Folkestad, B., Espehaug, B., Førland, O., and Aaslund, M.K. (2016) 'Predictors of outcomes following reablement in community-dwelling older adults', *Clinical Interventions in Aging*, 12: 55–63.

Vabø, M. and Szebehely, M. (2012) 'A caring state for all older people?', in A. Anttonen, L. Häikiö and K. Stefánsson (eds) *Welfare State, Universalism and Diversity*, Cheltenham: Edward Elgar, pp 121–43.

Vik, K. (2018) 'Hverdagsrehabilitering og tverrfaglig samarbeid; en empirisk studie i fire norske kommuner' ['Reablement and interprofessional collaboration; an empirical study in four Norwegian municipalities'], *Tidsskrift for omsorgsforskning* [*Journal of Care Reseach*], 4(1): 6-15.

Wærness, K. (1984) 'The rationality of caring', *Economic and Industrial Democracy*, 5(2): 185-211.

PART IV

Future perspectives

How can we help? Promoting autonomy-compatible help to reable older adults

Amy Clotworthy and Rudi Westendorp

Introduction: the current situation

As previous chapters of the book have addressed, the practice of reablement in many Western countries has developed primarily as a person-centred approach in response to a political need to adapt health- and social-care systems towards (expected) changes in the demographic composition of populations. In general, there has been a call for more holistic, integrated, and cost-effective approaches to long-term care provision – alternatives that enable a redistribution of resources, including financial means as well as professional workers to those who require complex care. At the same time, these new approaches should attempt to prevent unmet needs and care poverty elsewhere (see the introductory Chapter 1 by Rostgaard et al). In Chapters 3 and 4, the authors provided an overview of how the reablement paradigm has travelled and been implemented in parallel with developing ideas on 'successful ageing' and 'active and healthy citizens' in local and national practice, but also in relation to local 'bottom-up' initiatives and the agendas of supranational organisations. Although some scholars have concluded that 'reablement is a more effective rehabilitation service than traditional home-based services' for people with functional decline (for instance, Langeland et al, 2019), Chapter 5 by Lewin et al had discussed the lack of robust evidence for better client-level outcomes – perhaps also because reablement tends to be context-driven. However, as argued by Lewin et al, an approach that reduces the demand for aged-care services without negatively impacting individuals' health, functionality, and wellbeing may be a viable solution for ageing societies. At the same time, there may also be a need to re-focus the aims of reablement away from a preoccupation with reducing costs in the eldercare sector.

In order to prevent the collapse of the reablement movement due to not being (cost-)effective, we point to ways in which the ideals of the reablement paradigm could be better achieved in practice. Reablement is full of potential, and we hope it can avoid becoming a 'top–down', mechanical instrument only meant to benefit health economics.

The core of the 'reablement philosophy' refers to helping older people to do things for themselves rather than having things done for them (among others, Jones et al, 2009; Dahl et al, 2015; Clotworthy, 2020; Doh et al, 2019). Reablement's fundamental aim to provide this form of 'help to self-help' has also been linked to concepts like preventative care, rehabilitation, activation, and training (Dahl et al, 2015: 287). Because the reablement offer is also typically time-limited in many countries, the form of assistance being provided to older people has transitioned from long-term, compensating help to short-term, 'activating' support. As outlined in the book's introduction, a recent consensus among professionals defined reablement in part as 'a person-centred, holistic approach that aims to enhance an individual's physical and/or other functioning, to increase or maintain their independence in meaningful activities of daily living at their place of residence, and to reduce their need for long-term services' (Metzelthin et al, 2020: 11).

Despite the straightforward purpose of most reablement programmes, the international research in this area indicates that the concept of reablement lacks clarity both in theory and in practice, and there are inconsistencies in how it is defined and applied in specific contexts (Doh et al, 2019). Furthermore, most reablement programmes tend to reflect medical and psychological theories of successful ageing, and do not address sociocultural perspectives on ageing (Thuesen et al, 2021). This leads us to ask: could reablement programmes better recognise older people's intrinsic motivation, so they can reach their own self-identified goals, and more effectively achieve the programme's intended outcomes as expected from society? In this contribution, we first briefly examine the international research on reablement, starting from Doh et al's (2019) critical systematic review of the literature from 2005–2017. Using this review as a point of departure, we discuss what we believe is the central problem in the current reablement approach – specifically, a lack of focus on personal goals and intrinsic motivation, a notion that most studies overlook – and we then propose a new perspective that could significantly improve the practice with an emphasis on offering 'unhelpful help'.

State of the art: international research

In order to delineate some of reablement's common goals and features, Doh et al (2019) studied a range of reablement programmes being implemented worldwide. Based on how reablement was defined by leading scholars in the field (that is, 14 distinct definitions from 13 sources), the authors' review and analysis identified nine essential features of reablement: functionality, independence, short-term/time-limit, home and community setting, goal orientation, multidisciplinary team, a reduced need for ongoing support, social connectivity, and targeting. These features do not essentially deviate from the aforementioned Delphi study by Metzelthin et al (2020) in which 82 reablement experts from 11 countries aimed to develop a generally accepted definition of reablement.

In Doh et al's (2019) review, the most frequently cited feature of reablement was improving an older person's functionality (26 per cent), which referred to 'improving the ability of individuals to perform their daily living activities, and included therapies for increasing mobility (such as physiotherapy and occupational therapy) and cognition (such as stimulation exercises)' (Winkel et al, 2015; Aspinal et al, 2016; Legg et al, 2016; Vernooij-Dassen and Jeon, 2016; Tuntland, 2017, in Doh et al, 2019: 5). The next most-cited feature (15.2 per cent) was maximising independence, which is an expectation 'that reablement recipients will be able to do basic things for themselves, such as cooking, washing clothes, eating, using the toilet, grooming and bathing' (Doh et al, 2019: 6).

At the local level, reablement programmes typically employ an interdisciplinary team of physiotherapists and occupational therapists, registered nurses, homecare workers, and/or other paid staff (Cochrane et al, 2013; Aspinal et al, 2016; Tessier et al, 2016) who work specifically with participants age 65+. These older people may have already been receiving homecare services or recently been discharged from the hospital but, in many cases, reablement is not necessarily 'prompted by a specific acute event or illness but can also be implemented with people who have experienced a gradual decline in their health status and functioning' (Mishra and Barratt, 2016: 14). Thus, a primary aim of reablement is for older people to regain their skills in conducting activities of daily living (ADLs), such as preparing their own meals, bathing, dressing, and toileting, as well as managing instrumental activities of daily living (IADLs) that had previously been the remit of homecare service providers; for example, housekeeping, shopping, and managing medication. As such, a central goal of reablement is that older people 'will be more self-reliant and less dependent on help afterwards' (Rostgaard et al, 2016).

The unmet need: the watershed

Doh et al's (2019) critical review studied research on various reablement programmes being implemented worldwide. This review outlines several important strengths and weaknesses of reablement in terms of both meaning and practice. The authors' analysis of the literature raises many relevant points about functionality and social connectivity, and their proposed typology of four theoretical types of reablement suggests a way to improve overall outcomes. However, their conclusion fails to offer any specific suggestions for how to implement this typology in practice – or what the potential effect of doing so might be. Instead, the authors simply propose that reablement practitioners should shift their perspective to focus less on improving physical functionality and more on enhancing the ageing client's social connectivity within their homes and communities. Although this is a valid and important point, it seems to us that the authors have missed the underlying problem. Specifically, we believe that reablement professionals do need to change their focus and their perspective, but this requires a fundamental change in thinking and a commitment to move beyond certain professional paradigms.

There are ample descriptions of the prevailing health-economic driver 'that older adults' participation in reablement can improve functional outcomes for older people and has the potential to reduce their lifetime cost of care' (Francis et al, 2011; Tessier et al, 2016, in Doh et al, 2019: 2). This belief reflects an overall socio-political concern about the public-health challenges and potential economic burden posed by ageing populations, particularly the increased financial demands related to providing supportive health and welfare services for older people.

Reablement's biggest problems

As Doh et al's (2019) review indicates, many reablement programmes strongly emphasise improving an older person's physical functionality and independence – or helping them increase bodily competence and adapt to/ compensate for age-related changes in functional ability. Thus, part of the problem that has developed since the early 2000s seems to be that the concept of 'reablement' has become interchangeable with more standardised forms of physical rehabilitation, which tend to have a logical, linear approach to addressing disability and improving function through physical training and the use of adaptive equipment. In our evaluation of the literature (Clotworthy et al, 2021), reablement programmes have too often been implemented with an aim to reduce costs in the eldercare sector without emphasising the full scope of their potential beneficial effects and outcomes. In these goal-limited scenarios, physical and occupational therapy often include a specific form of clinical reasoning that is directed towards action (Mattingly, 1991: 981).

However, it should be emphasised that, even in this traditional way of working in which the professional uses 'narrative emplotment' – a central mode of clinical reasoning to determine the beginning, middle, and end of therapeutic training – both scholars and practitioners have stressed that these actions should be person-centred and incorporate shared decision-making (Mattingly, 1991: 982). This therapeutic practice is complex and interdependent, requiring continual reassessment and, as such, the overall process of rehabilitation must be continually adjusted and modified based on a person's physical, emotional, and ontological limitations, which are always in flux (Mattingly, 1991: 984). While it is generally impossible to know the outcome of any given course of physical rehabilitation due to these variables, it is often grounded in a professional approach that focuses on 'if this, then that'.

The pitfall that reablement professionals often face is approaching the older person's physical body as a site of potential; here, the 'if this, then that' outcome is that the older person should be able to embody (or re-embody) certain habits and competences. One of the meanings of 'potentiality' is 'a latent possibility imagined as open to choice, a quality perceived as available to human modification and direction through which people can work to propel an object or subject to become something other than it is' (Taussig et al, 2013:4), and research has described how this conceptualisation is often key to the professionals' approach (see Clotworthy, 2020). For example, in order to support older people in mastering meaningful daily activities so they can be as independent and self-helping as possible, some professionals tend to focus on improving 'muscle memory' through repetition so that the older person will remember specific movements, exercises, and instructions (Wolpert et al, 2001: 492). This may help to prevent falls and, more generally, to reduce fear and anxiety around performing actions that may put the ageing, injured, and/or ill body at risk (Clotworthy, 2020). However, reablement professionals often struggle to work with a corporeal body that is limited by pain, weakness, and a loss of function – and that, for a variety of reasons, may not always be able to 'remember' how to embody certain physical functions.

The key point about this approach is that the boundaries of both the problem that needs to be addressed and the most appropriate therapeutic training solution are more-or-less defined and fixed from the outset. In particular, we have observed that it is typically the professional who takes responsibility and assumes authority for defining the problem, the process, and how best to achieve the desired outcome. As a result, the roles of the professional and the older person are clearly separated, and the goal is simply to solve a specific problem (that the professional expert has defined). The danger, though, is that while many older people may indeed wish to improve their physical functionality and mobility to achieve greater independence both inside and outside the home (as well as to reduce risk), an over-emphasis on physical functionality instead reflects the 'comfort zone' of professionals.

Many contemporary reablement programmes mirror medical and psychological theories of successful ageing, including models of ageing that are associated with continuity, optimisation, selection, individuality, and goal-orientation, but most programmes do not address sociocultural perspectives on ageing (Thuesen et al, 2021). As older people experience physical functionality and the mastery of meaningful daily activities in a 'pertinent liminality within and between the sociocultural values of the third and fourth age' – that is, the transition from 'healthy-old' to disablement and dependency – it is important for reablement practitioners to consider the assumptions and underpinnings of current theories of ageing, and how they can help older people balance between optimising capacity and accepting the losses and limitations in their everyday lives (Thuesen et al, 2021).

In the transition from theory to policy and then to practice, we believe that reablement programmes tend to underemphasise older people's preferences and priorities with regards to being self-reliant and socially connected. A paternalistic approach in which the reablement team has the power to dictate the intended outcome of the service is contrary to the concepts of empowerment and intrinsic motivation that are key to achieving client-driven goals. This brings us from improving physical functionality and mastering meaningful daily activities to what we believe is the most important feature of reablement. In order to hone in on this feature, it is helpful to review the original conceptualisation of reablement.

Reablement's origin and its most essential feature

The fundamental principles of reablement have a long history (for an overview, see Clotworthy et al, 2021). For example, 'everyday rehabilitation' programmes began to be offered in Scandinavia in the 2000s. As presented in Chapters 2 and 3, the first was established in Östersund Municipality, Sweden, in 1999 and – inspired by the Swedes' positive experiences – soon began to develop in neighbouring Denmark in 2007 and Norway in 2012 (Clotworthy, 2020: 23); early experiences with the Scandinavian model were also communicated outside the scientific community (Ness and Horghagen, 2021). But the first widely disseminated reablement-related article was published in 2002, based on a US trial (Tinetti et al, 2002). Here, the authors described the essentials of a service model that was built on training relevant health professionals (that is, home care nurses, therapists, and home-health aides) as well as reorganising this home-care staff 'from individual care providers into an integrated, coordinated, interdisciplinary team with shared goals' (Tinetti et al, 2002: 2098). This required a 'reorientation of the focus of the home care team from primarily treating diseases and "taking care of" patients toward working together to maximize function and comfort' (Tinetti et al, 2002: 2098). This initiative had been developed based on findings from the researchers' earlier study, 'The design and implementation of a restorative care model for home care' (Baker et al, 2001) as well as previous research that examined older people's self-care and functionality with regards to performing meaningful activities of daily living in both hospital and home settings.

Tinetti et al wrote that the results of their trial suggested that 'reorganizing the structure and goals of home care holds promise for enhancing the functional and health outcomes of older persons' (Tinetti et al, 2002: 2104).

Most significantly, this early version of reablement was grounded in principles adapted from geriatric medicine, nursing, physical rehabilitation, and psychological goal-attainment; this refers to the belief that people 'are more likely to adhere to treatment plans if they are involved in setting goals and in determining the process for meeting these goals' (Tinetti et al, 2002: 2100). Thus, the initiative was grounded in 'the establishment of goals based on input from the patient, family, and home care staff, and agreement among this group on the process for reaching these goals' (Tinetti et al, 2002). From this description, we can clearly see that reablement was always meant to be different from standardised clinic-, hospital-, or even home-based physical rehabilitation.

Since then, reablement has seen a worldwide expansion, but, as we have suggested, some fundamental aspects seem to have fallen by the wayside. In terms of goal orientation, Doh et al's review found that there are 'systemic goals for reablement set by the sponsoring/funding body, such as reducing the need for ongoing support and cost containment' (2019: 8). Furthermore, 'the overall goal of reablement is the improved functionality and independence of clients. It follows that assessing individuals' progress on their personalised goals within a specified period is a key component of reablement practice (Miller, 2013), and presumably there are both short-term and long-term outcomes targeted for each client' (Doh et al, 2019: 8). Although personal goal-setting was considered to be important, it was not in all instances (Miller, 2013; Hjelle et al, 2017, in Doh et al, 2019: 7). The authors wrote that, when personal goal-setting is involved, it should focus on 'specific client needs and is driven by the client's aspirations and context' (Doh et al, 2019: 6); as such, reablement is 'person-centred (that is, directed towards the needs/wants of the individual clients, with involvement of clients in setting personalised goals for improving their functionality)' (Doh et al, 2019: 5).

Thus, in terms of how reablement programmes are organised, operationalised, and understood in practice, we argue that they should first and foremost recognise the heterogeneity of older people and support them in reaching their own *self-identified* goals. This is the original intent of reablement and undeniably its most essential feature. We question, however, whether the programmes that are currently being offered adequately support an older person's preferences and priorities; a statement that is underscored in Doh et al's review in which 'goal orientation' is only the fifth most-cited feature (10.9 per cent).

Why is goal orientation such a low priority in some settings? Our historical review of reablement programmes through time and space (Clotworthy et al, 2021) indicates that there may be a lack of capacity, training, and coordination/cohesion between professional groups to properly implement reablement services in practice; in particular, professional training, coordination, and compliance seem to remain problematic. Frequently, this is due to a lack of infrastructure, professional guidelines, training, and/or resources as well as an increased political drive to reduce the costs related to providing eldercare services. More to the point, it seems likely that reablement is 'nowhere near as effective as it could be' (Newton, 2012: 117) because it continues to lack personalisation and 'fails to appreciate what motivates people to make the substantial effort involved in regaining lost skills and abilities' (Newton, 2012: 117). We believe that a greater focus on personal goals and intrinsic motivation is precisely what is needed to ensure that reablement becomes a more supportive *and* a more effective initiative for older people worldwide.

Specific goals should be discussed and agreed upon early in the reablement trajectory in order to direct the course of training and to make explicit the older person's desired outcome. Various scholars have presented goal-planning as a relatively simple and straightforward way of interacting and subsequently prioritising the programme (as reviewed in Levack and Dean, 2012). However, other research, especially from New Zealand, suggests that the process of goal-setting often presents challenges, particularly with frail older people (Parsons et al, 2014). Moreover, the multiple approaches to goal-planning tend to involve a variety of procedures that may serve a range of different and often conflicting functions. Therefore, we suggest that professionals tailor their approach to the specific needs and priorities of each older person and, whenever possible, the objectives of their services should be based on relevant goal theory and current research (Levack and Dean, 2012).

It is often questioned whether reablement practices should be modified or whether outcomes vary among groups of people of different genders, race/ethnicity, socio-economic status, health status, and so on; there is very little data on these factors. This lack of evidence is generally considered a weakness of the current practice that should be addressed with specific research, trials, and stratified professional offerings. Given the core principle of reablement, however, we argue that services should be organised in accordance with goals that are meaningful to the individual, and are based on their specific personal context and environmental conditions – to a much higher degree than is the case today. In our view, any reference to the goals of specific groups or generalised strategies to achieve these aims is an infringement of reablement's core principle, and thereby increases the risk that reablement becomes entrenched as an instrumental and deterministic service.

Although Doh et al's (2019) typology of reablement calls for an emphasis on goal-setting in their professional focus, we believe that the authors have overlooked the essence of what is necessary to make reablement more effective in helping older people identify and achieve their own goals. In particular, we argue that there is a need for 'disruptive innovation' (Christensen et al, 2000) to effect substantial and meaningful change, and to ensure that older people's individual needs, priorities, and goals are acknowledged, heard, and supported. Specifically, we believe that there is a key logic at our fingertips that may help to make reablement more effective. It is a simple change in perspective but one that requires a paradigm shift: instead of focusing on set outcomes and economic benefits, professionals should 'help people help themselves' (Ellerman, 2001: ii) throughout the reablement trajectory. To provide some background for our proposal, we briefly describe philosopher David P. Ellerman's helping theory.

The solution: a focus on offering 'unhelpful help'

Reablement is meant to frame the older person as 'an expert in their own life' (Aspinal et al, 2016: 2; Rostgaard et al, 2016), and the health professionals' job is to find ways to help that individual remain independent and 'self-helping' for as long as possible. In their current iteration, reablement programmes point to the classic conundrum of trying to help people help themselves. Specifically, 'how can an outside party ("helper") assist those who are undertaking autonomous activities (the "doers") without overriding or undercutting their autonomy?' (Ellerman, 2001: ii). In his work for the United Nations Development Programme (UNDP)'s volume on *Capacity for Development*, Ellerman draws upon the fields of economics, management theory, psychology, sociology, mathematics, and philosophy to offer an analysis of why traditional forms of 'development assistance' are often inadequate and ineffective when provided to low-income countries.

In particular, Ellerman suggests that it is essential for humanitarian agencies and aid programmes to focus on 'autonomous self-development' whereby the professional helpers 'help in a way that respects, fosters, and sustains the autonomy of the doers' (Ellerman, 2005: 7). This means that any help given must be 'non-distortionary'; that is, the helping intervention should not 'change what the doer would do – given sufficient resources ... and does not distort the original motivation of the doer' (Ellerman, 2001: 2). This is similar to the principle of 'client self-determination', which is often applied in clinical practice and community care (Clark, 1998; Ragg, 2011: 29). This principle presumes that the people receiving help should make their own choices about how they want to live, and they should be given opportunities to take control of their own lives as much as possible. In this sense, they should be self-governing; that is, 'capable of choosing and responsible for their own lives, including their health-related behaviour' (Vallgårda, 2014: 341).

Ellerman recognises that helping people to help themselves is usually grounded in the work of certain professionals, and he points out that those who work in the 'helping professions' (for example, doctors, nurses, therapists, teachers, ministers, social workers, and so on) are in the 'paradoxical position of working to eliminate their own jobs' (Ellerman, 2005) in their efforts to support or enhance the self-reliant capacities of those they are trying to help. However, their work is more complex than that because the central problem is how to 'supply' help 'that actually furthers rather than overrides or undercuts the goal of the doers helping themselves' (Ellerman, 2005: 4). He states that autonomy – that is, the capacity of an agent to act – cannot be externally supplied. This means that, in providing help to promote greater independence and self-reliance, health professionals in particular cannot 'dictate values-driven outcomes without violating a core professional value' (Ragg, 2011: 29). Ellerman calls such supplied external motivation a 'direct or social engineering approach' (Ellerman, 2001: 5); these 'carrots and sticks' supply motivation by imposing conditionality, enforcing consequences for not reforming/complying, or providing incentives for failure. In other words, the 'Law of Unintended Rewards' (Murray, 1984: 212–15) becomes activated, wherein the doer may qualify for additional aid if they do not make certain behavioural changes the first time they are offered assistance. Ellerman writes that such supplied external motivations are most likely to produce 'cunning resistance rather than transformation' (Ellerman, 2001: 7).

Traditional forms of developmental aid and evidence-based-interventions in healthcare often contain a paternalistic approach; that is, they assume that experts can transfer essential information in an accurate and unbiased way so that individuals can be 'filled up (like an empty glass) with new knowledge and thereby transformed into informed and willing decision-makers' (Charles et al, 1999: 655). With this perspective, professional assistance from health experts is often meant to prevent 'negative' behaviours, such as developing a passive lifestyle after being diagnosed with a chronic disease (Dahl et al, 2015: 289). This approach also presumes that 'the professional knows best' – and indeed they might, but Ellerman insists that knowledge translation/ transfer is not the most effective way to instigate behaviour change that respects individual autonomy. Instead, he suggests a theory of 'unhelpful help' (Ellerman, 2005) – that is, professional judgement and assistance that is based on an individual's *intrinsic motivation*, and which is not open to intentional and deliberate choices. This is because this motivation comes from a person's unique sense of identity and history of lived experiences, which cannot be externally changed or acted upon. He states that the doers' actions 'will be guided by their knowledge, conceptual framework, values, and worldview, not those of the helpers' (Ellerman, 2001: 7). With this foundation in mind, Ellerman outlines a common framework for helpers trying to provide autonomy-compatible assistance to a particular set of doers:

- help must start from the present situation of the doers – not from a 'blank slate';
- helpers must see the situation through the eyes of the doers – not just through their own eyes;

- help cannot be imposed upon the doers – as that directly violates their autonomy;
- nor can doers receive help as a benevolent gift – as that creates dependency; and
- doers must be 'in the driver's seat' – which is the basic idea of autonomous self-direction. (Ellerman, 2001: ii)

In our opinion (and as Doh et al (2019) also suggest), reablement programmes tend to fall into several traps that contradict the idea of autonomy-compatible help. Many of these initiatives are designed to have a focus on person-centred goals and choices but, in practice, they may end up being more of a 'carrot and stick' intervention based on governments' economic ambitions to reduce long-term care costs and to prevent hospitalisation. Furthermore, by incorporating a 'closed-system' approach based on the health professional's authority, goals, and physical-training plans, reablement programmes may violate one of Ellerman's core tenets: 'helpers must see the situation through the eyes of the doers—not just through their own eyes'. However, it does not have to be this way. We believe that Ellerman's framework can help us 'correct' some of the missteps that contemporary reablement programmes seem to have been making. Next, we present an alternative conceptualisation of reablement as a programme that – rather than providing the more traditional form of 'help to self-help' to support functional ability and independence – emphasises offering 'unhelpful help' to promote self-choice and autonomy.

How can we promote autonomy-compatible reablement?

With regards to attaining a certain level of functional independence, scholars have earlier pointed out that there are risks in 'assuming any simple or standard concept of independence in the delivery of re-ablement services' (Wilde and Glendinning, 2012: 589). It is important to emphasise that, in many cultures and in many individual situations, older people themselves may not want to achieve independence – rather, this aim may come from the narrow focus of the health professionals. As such, a 'one size fits all' or outcome-driven approach to reablement will *always* be ineffective because humans are complex, irrational, and do not often conform to standardised models and operating logics; they are unable to deliver the 'right' results or achieve self-mastery on their own (Tronto, 2017: 31). Moreover, people need support and recognition from others; they become 'inter-dependent' in order to become socially connected and to make choices that will lead to meaningful action (Clotworthy, 2020). Thus, reablement should be an iterative, relational, social practice because, at the micro-level of everyday life, individual agency and autonomy can only emerge through interactional, social relationships (Clotworthy, 2020: 159). In a Swedish study that was conducted to illuminate older people's perceptions of a multi-professional team's caring skills as success factors for health support in short-term goal-directed reablement (Gustafsson et al, 2019), the authors concluded that health professionals' caring skills need to be addressed as an evidence base in the area of homecare for older people.

Thus, to more effectively engage older people in reablement, the health professional must first and foremost recognise the individual's self-identity and unique personhood. We believe that it is essential for the professional 'helpers' to focus on supporting the 'doer' in what they want to accomplish, and this form of autonomy-compatible help should be grounded in the doer's current needs and resources (physical, mental, and social) as well as their individual circumstances and personal desires. In this way, help starts 'from the present situation of the doers—not from a "blank slate"' (Ellerman, 2001: ii). By taking a point of departure in what an older person wants to achieve and gaining insight into the 'whole picture' of that unique person's life situation, the professional's main responsibility should be how to support the capacity of the agent to act – and not trying to provide 'managed knowledge' (Ellerman, 2001: 38). This means that, rather than a paternalistic, linear approach to knowledge translation and transfer or even a flexible training plan, the work of reablement should reflect a messy, 'open-system' approach that thrives on associative thinking, complexity, and a lack of focus on achieving a particular pre-defined outcome. Fundamentally, the health professional should focus on asking *why* – or even *whether* – it is important for the older person to participate in reablement, and then *listening* to their unique hopes and preferences.

We believe it is essential for the reablement professional to give the older person space to express these unique hopes and preferences, which form the basis of their intrinsic motivation. With this knowledge, the professional can then support the older person in determining the goals that are meaningful to them – goals which may or may not have anything to do with physical functionality, 'activities of daily living', or independence. When the doer defines both the problem and the desired outcome, they are *in the driver's seat*, assuming authority for and control of their reablement trajectory. The reablement professional should then allow the older person to determine which *meaningful* activities will make them feel more self-helping and competent in their everyday lives. The professional will also be able to guide the older person to discover new resources and activities that reflect their unique situation and what they ultimately want to achieve; such a sense of purpose promotes autonomy and social engagement, which may thereby have a positive impact on longevity and quality of life (Tomini et al, 2016; Pizzo, 2020).

In autonomy-compatible help, the roles of the helper and doer become interconnected with an emphasis on making shared decisions that simultaneously build learning capacity and support the older person's wishes, needs, and priorities. The use of a goal-facilitation tool in the assessment of an older person's needs during homecare has been shown to significantly improve outcomes as a consequence of individualised services tailored to the successful identification of the person's goals (Parsons and Parsons, 2012; Parsons et al, 2012). This is not an easy process and should not be restricted by time limits, which have been shown to have 'significant impacts on users' motivation and confidence to progress' (Wilde and Glendinning, 2012: 588). However, there may be a tension between how the reablement service is funded and the time needed to establish the older person's perspective on the purpose of the programme. Ideally, though, reablement programmes should be open-ended and defined by the doer, or possibly even blended into other care services.

Our proposal here may seem radical to governmental authorities who hope that time-limited reablement programmes can reduce the costs associated with their ageing populations. But we suggest that reablement should not focus on benchmarking progress, measuring outcomes, nor tracking physical milestones; most important, it should not be framed in cost-savings or economic terms, such as a 'return on investment'. Instead, reablement must focus on *people* – it should be an offer that supports older people in building their resources and enhancing their social connectivity, which has a markedly positive effect on overall health, wellbeing, and longevity (Tomini et al, 2016; Pizzo, 2020). In the messy, 'open-system' approach we are advocating here, it should not be up to the helper – either a government entity or a family member or a health professional – to determine the doer's goals and needs, or how best to improve their quality of life. Quite simply, reablement professionals should not impose help upon the doers by emplotting a rehabilitation plan and saying, 'Here's how I can help you become more self-helping'. Instead, they should simply ask the older person, 'What matters to you, and how can I help you achieve your goals?' And then listen – *really listen* – to the answer.

Final reflections

Our proposal may lead readers to ask: how can this new approach to reablement work in a world of increasing fiscal and organisational constraints? Where can we find inspiration for a new way forward that will further develop and refine current reablement models? One initiative that should be considered is the Dutch homecare provider called *Buurtzorg* ('neighbourhood care'). First developed in 2006, this nurse-led form of holistic care has revolutionised community care in the Netherlands, and it is now expanding into many other countries worldwide. For instance, in Denmark, one local version of the model was launched as 'Coffee first' to emphasise the need to get to know the older person and their personal situation before planning how to help them. The Buurtzorg model is grounded in 'the client perspective and then works outwards to assemble solutions that bring independence and improved quality of life' (Buurtzorg, 2021); in particular, this direct-care approach focuses on the client's 'living environment, the people around the client, a partner or relative at home, and on into the client's informal network; their friends, family, neighbours and clubs as well as professionals already known to the client in their formal network' (Buurtzorg, 2021). A key element of the model is that the health professional must have 'a sustained focus on the opportunities (in care as well as the local community) that exist to support the citizen's autonomy and self-help' (Gray et al, 2015); as such, the Buurtzorg approach is meant to provide the greatest possible continuity in care as well as a starting point for an ongoing and holistic approach to the citizen's need for help (Buch, 2020: 20). In the Buurtzorg model, we can recognise the messy, 'open-system' approach that we have described previously – in particular, the lack of focus on achieving a particular pre-defined outcome gives control back to the ageing adult.

Although experiences in other countries have raised questions regarding 'the applicability and relevance of the model within different cultural contexts and the potential of the model to produce both local and global impact' (Kreitzer et al, 2015: 44), the significance of the Buurtzorg concept may ultimately lie 'not just in the wholesale spread of this model but in the recognition of the value of its key components' (Gray et al, 2015: 6). Specifically, founder Jos de Blok has said that Buurtzorg is 'a company that is driven by a belief in "humanity over bureaucracy," and that belief deeply impacts the patients and those who care for them' (Kreitzer et al, 2015: 40). Putting economic markets and organisational ambitions before people's needs and priorities can be problematic, as it erodes trust between the professional and the client; the result is that, instead of maximising their (learning) abilities, the older person's resources become suppressed.

In line with Buurtzorg, we argue that – both fundamentally and on a higher, societal level – government officials and health professionals should focus less on trying to improve older persons' functional ability in order to train these individuals to be 'free' from the need for health and welfare services. Rather than the current focus on productivity, cost-savings, and independence that has become a central driver of many reablement programmes worldwide, government officials and health professionals should put more effort into building stronger, more inclusive communities of care (Clotworthy, 2020: 222). Such communities would include institutional infrastructures that acknowledge and value human complexity – that is, irrationality, limitations, and 'messy' systems. They would also promote inclusion and reflect a variety of sociocultural perspectives on ageing

(Thuesen et al, 2021). But most essential, such communities of care would include health professionals who are able to help older people 'balance between optimising capacity and accepting losses in their everyday life' (Moe and Brinchmann, 2016; Thuesen et al, 2021: 1); this perspective would help them to make sense of their change in functionality, and thereby allow them to articulate a new sense of self (Mattingly, 1991). In this way, older people would be able 'to pursue their dreams and live their lives as they wish' (Yglesias, 2015). With a foundation in complexity and a messy, 'open-system' approach that supports older people's intrinsic motivation and self-identified goals, reablement programmes would be more effective and would *also* enhance older people's autonomy and social engagement; this in turn would improve their quality of life and reaffirm their value as important members of society.

References

Aspinal, F., Glasby, J., Rostgaard, T., Tuntland, H., and Westendorp, R. (2016) 'New horizons: reablement – supporting older people towards independence', *Age and Ageing*, 45(5): 574–8.

Baker, D.I., Gottschalk, M., Eng, C., Weber, S., and Tinetti, M.E. (2001) 'The design and implementation of a restorative care model for home care', *The Gerontologist*, 41(2): 257–63.

Buch, M.S. (2020) *Buurtzorgs model for hjemmesygepleje og hjemmepleje – Introduktion til modellen, oversigt over litteraturen og perspektiver for afprøvninger i en dansk kontekst* [*Buurtzorg's Model for Home Nursing and Home Care – Introduction to the Model, Overview of the Literature, and Perspectives on Trials in a Danish Context*]. Copenhagen: VIVE [online], Available from: https://pure.vive.dk/ws/files/4552337/301713_Buurtzorgs_model_for_hjemmesyge pleje_og_hjemmepleje_PDU_UA.pdf.

Buurtzorg (2021) 'Buurtzorg's model of care' [online], Available from: https://www.buurtzorg.com/about-us/buurtzorgmodel/

Charles, C., Gafni, A., and Whelan, T. (1999) 'Decision-making in the physician–patient encounter: revisiting the shared treatment decision-making model', *Social Science & Medicine*, 49: 651–61.

Christensen, C.M., Bohmer, R., and Kenagy, J. (2000) 'Will disruptive innovations cure health care?', *Harvard Business Review*, September/October: 102–17 [online], Available from: http://achc.org.co/hospital 360/propuesta/Sincronizacion/Tecnologia_Disruptiva/Innovaciones_disr uptivas.pdf.

Clark, C. (1998) 'Self-determination and paternalism in community care: practice and prospects', *The British Journal of Social Work*, 28(3): 357–402.

Clotworthy, A. (2020) *Empowering the Elderly? How "Help to Self-help" Interventions Shape Ageing and Eldercare in Denmark*, Bielefeld, Germany: transcript Verlag.

Clotworthy, A., Kusumastuti, S., and Westendorp, R. (2021) 'Reablement through time and space: a scoping review of how the concept of "reablement" for older people has been defined and operationalised', *BMC Geriatrics*, 21(61): 1–16.

Cochrane, A., McGilloway, S., Furlong, M., Molloy, D., and Stevenson, M. (2013) 'Home-care "re-ablement" services for maintaining and improving older adults' functional independence', *Cochrane Database of Systematic Reviews*, Issue 11, Art. No.: CD010825. DOI: 10.1002/14651858. CD010825

Dahl, H.M., Eskelinen, L., and Hansen, E.B. (2015) 'Coexisting principles and logics of elder care: Help to self-help and consumer-oriented service?', *International Journal of Social Welfare*, 24: 287–95.

Doh, D., Smith, R., and Gevers, P. (2019) 'Reviewing the reablement approach to caring for older people', *Ageing & Society*, 40(6): 1371–83.

Ellerman, D. (2001) 'Helping people help themselves: towards a theory of autonomy-compatible help', Policy Research Working Paper 2693, Washington, DC: World Bank. DOI: 10.1596/1813-9450-2693

Ellerman, D. (2005) *Helping People Help Themselves: From the World Bank to an Alternative Philosophy of Development Assistance*, Ann Arbor, MI: University of Michigan Press.

Francis, J., Fisher, M., and Rutter, D. (2011) *Reablement: A Cost-effective Route to Better Outcomes*, London: Social Care Institute for Excellence.

Gray, B.H., Sarnak, D.O., and Burgers, J.S. (2015) 'Home care by self-governing nursing teams: The Netherlands' Buurtzorg model', The Commonwealth Fund, 29 May [online], Available from: https://www.commonwealthfund.org/publications/case-study/2015/may/home-care-self-governing-nursing-teams-netherlands-buurtzorg-model

Gustafsson, L.-K., Östlund, G., Zander, V., Elfström, M.L., and Anbäcken, E.-M. (2019) '"Best fit" caring skills of an interprofessional team in short-term goal-directed reablement: older adults' perceptions', *Scandinavian Journal of Caring Sciences*, 33(2): 498–506.

Hjelle, K.M., Tuntland, H., Førland, O., and Alvsvåg, H. (2017) 'Driving forces for home-based reablement: a qualitative study of older adults' experiences', *Health & Social Care in the Community*, 25(5): 1581–9.

Jones, K.C., Baxter, K., Curtis, L.A., Arksey, H., Forder, J.E., Glendinning, C., and Rabiee, P. (2009) 'Investigating the longer term impact of home care re-ablement services: the short-term outcomes and costs of home care re-ablement services', Working Paper DHR 2378. Social Policy Research Unit, University of York, October [online], Available from: https://www.york.ac.uk/inst/spru/research/pdf/ReablementOutcomes.pdf.

Kreitzer, M.J., Monsen, K.A., Nandram, S., and de Blok, J. (2015) 'Buurtzorg Nederland: a global model of social innovation, change, and whole-systems healing', *Global Advances in Health and Medicine*, 4(1): 40–4.

Langeland, E., Tuntland, H., Folkestad, B., Førland, O., Jacobsen, F.F., and Kjeken, I. (2019) 'A multicenter investigation of reablement in Norway: a clinical controlled trial', *BMC Geriatrics*, 19(29). DOI: 10.1186/ s12877-019-1038-x

Legg, L., Gladman, J., Drummond, A., and Davidson, A. (2016) 'A systematic review of the evidence on home care reablement services', *Clinical Rehabilitation*, 30(8): 741–9.

Levack, W. and Dean, S.G. (2012) 'Processes in rehabilitation', in S.G. Dean, R.J. Siegert, and W.T. Taylor (eds) *Interprofessional Rehabilitation: A Person-Centred Approach*, West Sussex, UK: John Wiley & Sons.

Mattingly, C. (1991) 'What is clinical reasoning?', *American Journal of Occupational Therapy*, 45(11): 979–86.

Metzelthin, S., Rostgaard, T., Parsons, M., and Burton, E. (2020) 'Development of an internationally accepted definition of reablement: a Delphi study', *Ageing and Society*, 42(3): 703–18.

Miller, E. (2013) 'Embedding outcomes in the reablement model in North Lanarkshire', Glasgow: Economic and Social Research Council, University of Strathclyde, October [online], Available from: http://www.reablement. it/sites/default/files/pdf/outcomes-in-reablement-report-full.pdf

Mishra, V. and Barratt, J. (2016) *Reablement and Older People* [online], Available from: http://www.ifa-copenhagen-summit.com/wp-content/ uploads/2016/04/Copenhagen-Summit-Final-Report.pdf

Moe, C. and Brinchmann, B.S. (2016) 'Optimising capacity – a service user and caregiver perspective on reablement', *Grounded Theory Review*, 15: 25–40.

Murray, C. (1984) *Losing Ground: American Social Policy, 1950–1980*, New York: Basic Books.

Ness, N.E. and Horghagen, S. (2021) 'Occupational therapy in Norway: influence of the Nordic welfare state policy and the professional development of occupational therapy and occupational science worldwide', *Annals of International Occupational Therapy*, 4(1). DOI: 10.3928/ 24761222-20200413-04

Newton, C. (2012) 'Personalising reablement: inserting the missing link', *Working with Older People*, 16(3): 117–21.

Parsons, J.G.M. and Parsons, M.J.G. (2012) 'The effect of a designated tool on person-centred goal identification and service planning among older people receiving homecare in New Zealand', *Health & Social Care in the Community*, 20(6): 653–62.

Parsons, J.G.M., Rouse, P., Robinson, E.M., Sheridan, N., and Connolly, M.J. (2012) 'Goal setting as a feature of homecare services for older people: does it make a difference?', *Age & Ageing*, 41(1): 24–9.

Parsons, J.G.M., Jacobs, S., and Parsons, M.J.G. (2014) 'The use of goals as a focus for services for community dwelling older people', in R.J. Siegert and W. Levack (eds) *Handbook of Rehabilitation Goal Setting*, San Francisco: CRC Press/Taylor & Francis.

Pizzo, P.A. (2020) 'A prescription for longevity in the 21st century: renewing purpose, building and sustaining social engagement, and embracing a positive lifestyle', *Journal of the American Medical Association*, 323(5): 415–16.

Ragg, D.M. (2011) *Developing Practice Competencies: A Foundation for Generalist Practice*, Hoboken, NJ: Wiley.

Rostgaard, T., Aspinal F., Glasby, J., Tuntland, H., and Westendorp, R. (2016) *Reablement*, Copenhagen: KORA Publications.

Taussig, K.-S., Høyer, K., and Helmreich, S. (2013) 'The anthropology of potentiality: an introduction to Supplement 7', *Current Anthropology*, 54(S7): S3–14.

Tessier, A., Beaulieu, M.-D., Mcginn, C.A., and Latulippe, R. (2016) 'Efficacit é de l'autonomisation: une revue systématique' ['Effectiveness of reablement: a systematic review'], *Politiques de sante* [*Healthcare Policy*], 11(4): 49–59.

Thuesen, J., Feiring, M., Doh, D., and Westendorp, R. (2021) 'Reablement in need of theories of ageing: would theories of successful ageing do?', *Ageing & Society*, 1–13. DOI: 10.1017/S0144686X21001203

Tinetti, M.E., Baker, D., Gallo, W.T., Nanda, A., Charpentier, P., and O'Leary, J. (2002) 'Evaluation of restorative care vs usual care for older adults receiving an acute episode of home care', *Journal of the American Medical Association*, 287(16): 2098–105.

Tomini, F., Tomini, S.M., and Groot, W. (2016) 'Understanding the value of social networks in life satisfaction of elderly people: a comparative study of 16 European countries using SHARE data', *BMC Geriatrics*, 16(203). DOI: 10.1186/s12877-016-0362-7

Tronto, J. (2017) 'There is an alternative: homines curans and the limits of neoliberalism', *International Journal of Care and Caring*, 1(1): 27–43.

Tuntland, H., Kjeken, I., Langeland, E., Folkestad, B., Espehaug, B., Førland, O., and Aaslund, M.K. (2017) 'Predictors of outcomes following reablement in community-dwelling older adults', *Clinical Interventions in Ageing*, 12: 55–63.

Vallgårda, S. (2014) 'Ethics, equality and evidence in health promotion: Danish guidelines for municipalities', *Scandinavian Journal of Public Health*, 42(4): 337–43.

Vernooij-Dassen, M. and Jeon, Y.-H. (2016) 'Social health and dementia: the power of human capabilities', *International Psychogeriatrics*, 28(5): 701–3.

Wilde, A. and Glendinning, C. (2012) '"If they're helping me then how can I be independent?" The perceptions and experience of users of home-care re-ablement services', *Health & Social Care in the Community*, 20: 583–90.

Winkel, A., Langberg, H., and Wæhrens, E.E. (2015) 'Reablement in a community setting', *Disability and Rehabilitation*, 37(15): 1347–52.

Wolpert, D.M., Ghahramani, Z., and Flanagan, J.R. (2001) 'Perspectives and problems in motor learning', *Trends in Cognitive Sciences*, 5(11): 487–94.

Yglesias, M. (2015). 'Denmark's Prime Minister says Bernie Sanders is wrong to call his country Socialist', *Vox*, 31 October [online], Available from: https://www.vox.com/2015/10/31/9650030/denmark-prime-minister-bernie-sanders

11

A cross-country reflection on empirical and theoretical learnings, challenges, and the way forward for reablement

John Parsons, Hanne Tuntland, Michelle Nelson,
Rudi Westendorp, and Tine Rostgaard

Introduction

The book has provided an interdisciplinary, comparative, as well as a critical investigation of reablement practice, investigating reablement from the perspectives of research, theory, and practice. In this concluding chapter, we want to take the opportunity to reflect on the content of the book chapters, and with a focus on the convergence/divergence of reablement tracks, the challenges and learnings, as well as the implications for theory, practice and policy-making.

The chapter has been developed following a facilitated online discussion between five members of the ReAble Network and based on a reading of all chapters. The participants in the discussion were: Tine Rostgaard (Professor, Stockholm University, Sweden, and Roskilde University, Denmark); Hanne Tuntland (Professor, Western Norway University of Applied Sciences and Associate Professor, Oslo Metropolitan University, Norway); Rudi Westendorp (Professor, University of Copenhagen, Denmark); Michelle Nelson (Assistant Professor, University of Toronto, Canada); and John Parsons (Associate Professor, The University of Auckland, New Zealand). The discussion was structured around a number of key questions and was recorded and transcribed.

The chapter summarises the key learnings and messages from the book and, using quotes from the discussion, illustrates the potential implications for reablement practice and research. Moreover, the editors reflect in the conclusion over the key issues discussed in the book, learning points and the way forward.

What is the main message of the book?

The first question posed to the five participants in the facilitated discussion related to what they believed was the main message of the book. It was here acknowledged that the contributors to the book are from nine countries across three continents and represent various disciplinary backgrounds. Most of the chapters have a cross-country and cross-disciplinary comparative perspective. In addition, the combination of both a researcher's and a clinician's perspective are of particular note:

'The book brings together two different perspectives. It's one of the health professionals who analyses the implications for clinical practice and client-level outcomes. The other perspective is from social scientists who analyse the political possibilities and constraints within the service delivery situation.'

Furthermore, basing the book on the ReAble Network of international collaborators was seen as a strength of the book, which allowed the identification of key messages relating to the development and implementation of reablement across the participating countries.

'I think having a network that was structured around a topic that was international and then working to produce a product required us to dig in and discuss, determine where we had conceptual alignment ... We don't necessarily in our different jurisdictions see all the same way. This required us to say: 'OK, well, what's different in Norway versus Canada versus New Zealand?'. That if we are reflective of the kind of the knowledge base of our country, of our jurisdiction, what's at play? And I think it gave us an academic and a practice perspective to explore the concept from.'

What is the purpose of reablement?

In 2016, Legg et al noted that reablement is an ill-defined intervention, targeting an ill-defined patient population. In response, Metzelthin et al (2020) conducted a Delphi-based consensus definition of reablement, also presented in Chapter 1 by Rostgaard et al. In many cases, this book has a central focus on the Delphi definition of reablement, which proposes that the purpose of reablement is to enhance an individual's physical and/ or other functioning, and to increase or maintain their independence in meaningful activities of daily living. The facilitated discussion dealt with what reablement entails, and whether the boundaries of what reablement is, should be expanded.

The participants in the discussion agreed that the Delphi study is helpful for reaching an agreement on the characteristics, components, aims, and target groups of reablement. However, the current definition could best be described as a conceptual definition and there is an ongoing need for the development of an operational definition also. Such a definition may support the transferability of evidence between heterogeneous settings and services, a lack of which has been a criticism of reablement research. Consideration of the Delphi definition and its limitations prompted a discussion of the philosophical underpinnings of the Delphi consensus definition and the need to consider its further development.

'The [Delphi] definition is conceptual but not operational. I wondered if the operationalisation of the definition requires some further discussion to support transferability between settings and contexts. I think we have an obligation, though, to show the kind of blurry edge where if there is the potential to extend or refine our definition based on emerging work, and not close it out to say because it doesn't fit our current definition of reablement. That emphasises the importance of the theoretical foundation of the work and making that explicit. The current definition of reablement has a particular philosophical foundation. This text, and within our network, is a place where we actually make that explicit as well so that people can agree or disagree or critique current work.'

This highlights the potential need for context-bound national definitions that use the basis of the context-free Delphi definition. In this way, reablement will have the key components common to the Delphi definition but with an additional focus that ensures that the local contextual variations are able to be considered.

The focus of reablement

There was considerable discussion about the difference in the focus and target of reablement services. Targeting older people who have experienced recent functional decline is a common focus in reablement across countries, and this is reflected in the available published research. However, there are examples where reablement does not have this focus. For example, Chapter 8 by Rahja and Thuesen illustrates that reablement service models have been adapted to support people with long-standing needs, such as those with dementia.

Some of the authors of this concluding chapter felt that reablement is a rehabilitation service and that the target group is indeed people with functional decline; as such, the therapy needs to focus on enhancing some kind of functioning. However, in Chapter 10, Clotworthy and Westendorp argue that this is a relatively narrow focus on reablement. They present findings reported in the international literature that, when implementing the reablement paradigm, the programs sometimes lose sight of their overall purpose, which the authors state is to support older people's preferences with regards to being self-reliant, independent and socially connected. In particular, Clotworthy and Westendorp argue that there may be too much emphasis in policy and practice on physical functioning at a cost of ignoring social connectivity and/or wellbeing. This tension was also apparent in the facilitated discussion with the identification of the need for a holistic view of the scope of reablement services rather than a focus on physical rehabilitation with tangible outcomes. This discord is present across a number of the book chapters and is an important issue to consider in the aim, design, delivery, and evaluation of reablement services. This consideration may well involve the fundamental policy principle driving the delivery of reablement within a country, region, or jurisdiction. Chapter 3 by Feiring et al highlights the variation in the application of the international rhetorical frames of healthy and active ageing across UK, Australasia, and Scandinavia. Within these regions there is a discourse that may prioritise a focus on self-reliance and independence as outcomes of reablement service provision in order to make long-term care systems more financially sustainable in an ageing world. However, as also noted in the book, this rhetorical frame sits within a particular sociocultural understanding of ageing which is indeed not universal. Also, it carries with it the risk that reablement becomes too focused on the production of functioning, rather than being.

There was also considerable discussion of the liminal nature of reablement where services are often not solely offered in a health or a social-care setting, but often try to bridge the best of both. The participants felt that this needed to be acknowledged and considered when designing and evaluating reablement service models. In addition, the liminal position of many older people when they commence reablement services was seen as a key feature that needed to be considered in the design and content of services. This is considered in an article by Thuesen et al (2021), co-authored by one of the participants in the discussion.

'I think the older people who are users of reablement services are often in that liminal space. They've lived their life and suddenly they have maybe an acute event, or maybe it's a slow deterioration that has prompted a referral to reablement services. I don't think as service providers, as clinicians, we respond particularly well to that. Reablement services often focus on improving function or maintaining function, not actually having the conversation with the older person and their family. "You know, you may not regain your function. This may be what your life is going to look like".'

The promotion of opportunities for debate and discussion of these foundations was seen as central to the evolution and expansion of reablement. The need for an acknowledgement of the competing imperatives and purposes of reablement should be clearly identified, together with the theoretical aspects of reablement at a grand-, meta-, mid-, and micro-range level. These theoretical aspects are described in Chapter 2 by Tuntland et al, and consider the wider perspective of the fundamental theoretical foundations of reablement. At a grand-level theory, both the system and the community perspective on the dominant paradigm that drives health and social care are included. The meta-range level of theory considers theories relating to ageing. At a mid-range level, theories that help to understand what drives and motivates users of reablement services are included, whereas at a micro-range level, relevant theories for reablement explore change mechanisms as to how and why interventions have an impact on the individual client.

Commonalities across countries in idea – but variation in implementation of reablement

The need to identify and resolve any areas where the practice of reablement differed across a country or jurisdiction was seen as something that was important to the ongoing development and refinement of reablement. Furthermore, there was an acknowledgement that countries – despite different approaches to the organisation of long-term care – face similar challenges when implementing reablement. These include challenges at the level of funding, staffing, and also in engaging with older people and their families. These concepts are explored across the chapters in this book and illustrate the importance of a focus on acknowledgement of the impact of the features of a reablement model when designing and delivering services. Once more, the need for clarity of purpose, an acknowledgement of the fundamental features of reablement, and a recognition of the requirement to allow for the influence of the local context were considered in the discussion to be important. This was highlighted further in comments about the different book chapters that illustrate the need for a tailored response that meets the needs in the particular country.

> 'I think we have an interesting chapter, the travelling [Chapter 3 by Feiring et al], which shows the yes, how the idea travels between countries and very different [welfare] contexts, and where the different actual groups shape the different agendas, and therefore create and develop different models. We can all see the idea behind the philosophy [of reablement], but the actual practice and how it's implemented might differ. We also see that in Chapter 4 by Parsons et al, I think very well.

So yes, the context matters very much [to the way that reablement is planned and implemented].'

Reablement research

The issue of research relating to reablement is the focus of considerable content within this book. The facilitated discussion further explored the relationship between the competing philosophical foundations of reablement and the often contradictory evidence generated by single studies and systematic reviews.

'When you look at the user perspective, we have qualitative research which has shown service users are very satisfied with reablement. In particular, I think that clients who are frail, have mobility issues and balance issues [benefit] from reablement. And when they have reablement care workers at their side, in their homes or in their community, they do tasks for the first time after recovering from hospital. It may be the first time they climb stairs, the first time they take the bus, then they dare to take risk with people present. If not having a reablement care worker present, they would be more passive, not active participants in their own life. In addition, research regarding effectiveness has shown that in the short term, in a six-month perspective, clients function better in daily activities, they improve their physical functioning and also health-related quality of life. So yes, they benefit from reablement. And that's our research findings – however, not much supported by systematic reviews so far.'

The tension to demonstrate effectiveness within the robust constraints of a systematic review was highlighted. This, once more, relates to the need for further clarity around the purpose and key features of reablement, including the optimal group to target with reablement services. But the participants also reflected on whether such evaluation methods are too rigid for interventions like reablement which differ according to the client's aims and goals.

'The problem with reablement that is often coming up in the systematic reviews is that we can't prove that it works because ... we've tried to apply it across different settings, and that makes it hard to define it in a quantifiable manner. And so, I think the book has teased out the issue that if we work in an evidence-based health care system where we need to demonstrate reductions in cost, reduction in health care utilisation, cost–utility, that's hard to do. If we look at the way that we implement reablement services – and I think this comes up in a couple of the chapters – it's hard to quantify because it is so context-driven.'

A central message of the book is that there is a need to broaden the focus of reablement research to not only consider effectiveness in improving user outcomes and managing costs. The inclusion of robust process evaluation that explores the detail of what is delivered as well as the intensity of services should be a parallel stream of research relating to reablement studies. Alongside this, there are opportunities for implementation-evaluation methods to be incorporated into future research to further define the contextual factors that seem to influence outcomes resulting from reablement. This is highlighted in the Buma et al (2022) systematic review who suggest that there need to be three key areas of focus in reablement research. First, there needs to be a clearer description of the content of reablement interventions, with intervention publication of protocols that make use of valid reporting guidelines and the use of process evaluations to assess the variation in results of effect studies. Second, through the use of networking opportunities, such as the ReAble Network, there needs to be additional input from reablement experts, who have developed, evaluated, and implemented reablement interventions. Such data should be used to develop and evaluate reablement interventions. Lastly, there is a need for more high-quality studies of reablement using outcomes to identify reablement model features that are more promising than others, and investigate which combination of features is most effective.

Moreover, researchers should consider the need for a common definition of reablement to allow for direct comparison across studies. The use of process evaluation and other similar methods would then enable a more nuanced consideration of where reablement service provision may differ across contexts/studies.

An ongoing focus on integrating the voice of the older person and their family is important to consider in future research and is a way to ensure that the developing evidence for reablement is congruent to the needs and values of the users of the service. This focus would align to the key message in Chapter 10 by Clotworthy and Westendorp.

In addition, the potential impact of reablement on perceptions and experiences of staff, as outlined in Chapter 9 by Rostgaard and Graff, is another issue to consider. The discussion participants considered this exploration of the wider effect of reablement across time and sectors to be a vital next step in evaluating the effects of reablement.

Another area that needs consideration in future research relates to the long-term effects of reablement, particularly as a whole system approach that includes the impact on health and social care outcomes as well as its impact at a family/individual level. This is highlighted by the conclusion in Chapter 5 by Lewin et al that questions whether a lack of robust evidence for better client-level outcomes should influence the adoption of reablement into a service system. The authors suggest that with the developing evidence of positive impact on health and wellbeing and quality of life, there is also in these times of population ageing, a need for an approach that reduces the demand for aged care services and does not negatively impact on individuals' health, function, and wellbeing, is surely a better use of public money than one which will need ever-increasing funding as demand is fuelled by increasing numbers of older people.

Lessons learnt about reablement

The discussion about the published evidence involving reablement prompted a close consideration of a key theme presented within the book: that a common alignment of ideas has led many countries to implement reablement (as illustrated in both Chapter 3 by Feiring et al and Chapter 4 by Parsons et al). However, the complexity of implementing reablement within a country or region necessitates a very considered approach to defining, designing, delivering, and evaluating the service. The participants in the discussion hope that the content of this book will support practitioners, policy makers, and researchers to identify the key features that they need to consider in their local context.

Another discussion point related to the need to consider the cultural context when implementing a new service such as reablement. There is an acknowledgment that reablement has only rarely been implemented outside of high-income countries in the US, Europe, and Australasia. Further, there has been little focus on how reablement aligns with cultural values and beliefs of minority ethnic groups within these countries, where health and wellbeing may be conceptualised in quite different ways.

'To this point, most of the implementation [of reablement] has been in quite individualist countries, such as New Zealand, with a Māori [indigenous people of New Zealand] population, which is far more collectivist. And so often older Māori do not see the point of doing something that is focused on their health and wellbeing as the focus should be on the health and wellbeing of the wider group. This point of doing something for their partner or their wider family, of which they are a part, and so often they will prioritise their whanau [extended family's] needs over their own individual things. This is also something I have observed working with other cultures, including older Chinese people with really strong beliefs about filial piety. The respect for elders among the family often means that you don't make them struggle to do stuff.'

The issue of funding models for reablement was also an issue that was highlighted as being a key learning point. Some countries focus on funding as a strategy to drive behaviour and change within reablement service provision.

'One of the most important learnings in New Zealand, was that [the system] really struggled with reablement until the funding model was changed. It was realised that paying for reablement on a unit level, paying for hours, and paying for inputs didn't foster a culture in organisations that actually responded to the needs identified by the older person in their family. And so, changing the funding to a needs-based case-mix model really allowed the flexibility.'

Conclusions and the way forward

This book has presented a critical investigation of reablement in an interdisciplinary and international context to enable the development of new knowledge and understanding of this complex intervention. The experience presented from the countries where reablement has been delivered and evaluated over the past two decades clearly demonstrates that reablement is at a critical point in terms of ongoing development and refinement. The most pressing issue that needs to be considered and resolved relates to the fundamental questions of what reablement is and how it is used.

Reablement has developed from the concepts of active and healthy ageing with a strong influence from fundamental rehabilitation principles, theories, and concepts. The developing evidence demonstrates that reablement has a positive impact on a number of key outcomes at the level of those who both receive and deliver reablement. In addition, the effect of reablement on providing sustainable and high-quality services to vulnerable groups and within the current resource capacity has been established. Furthermore, the critical components of reablement service delivery models have been identified, and include a focus on individualised and person-centred assessment and intervention, a trained and experienced interdisciplinary team and an organisational model that enables the funding and other resources necessary. However, there are considerable challenges and opportunities relating to the use of reablement in the near future.

First, reablement has been successfully implemented regardless of differences in welfare and long-term care systems. However, the potential for the use of reablement outside of high-income countries is uncertain. The countries considered in this book have well developed long-term care systems with considerable use of highly trained physiotherapy, occupational therapy, and nursing resources located within community settings. It is unclear how reablement models would need to be refined in order to be used in low-income countries. In addition, there is a clear need to look at the potential use of reablement among other groups that have not been a focus to this point. This may include a consideration of cultural diversity to ensure the alignment with beliefs and values relating to health and wellbeing of all cultural groups. Furthermore, the exciting and developing focus on designing and delivering reablement services that target specific groups such as those with dementia has considerable potential to provide individually tailored support that achieves meaningful outcomes.

A further consideration at the practice level relates to the reablement care worker. The book chapters present a compelling case for the importance of a focus on training of reablement team members, and the impact of the interdisciplinary team on successful outcomes. However, there is a clear need to support and consider the views and experience of reablement care workers.

A key learning point from both the book content and the experience across a number of countries in recent years is that there is an identified need to critically reflect on fundamental beliefs and values of reablement and to ensure that there is adequate consideration of the theoretical assumptions. This includes critical reflection on the common focus of reablement practice towards physical functionality rather than on social connectivity. Furthermore, greater consistency is needed within the evaluation of reablement models with an identified need to agree on the required outcomes for reablement. There is also a need to consider the meaning of the developing evidence base relating to reablement. At the client-level and the cost-effectiveness level, the evidence is mixed with a clear need for more high quality studies.

Finally, there is a real risk that municipalities or jurisdictions gradually diminish reablement service models to a light version of reablement in order to reduce costs. However, if reablement is not person-centred, multimodal, intensive, and with a breadth of professions, it is unknown whether the intervention is still effective.

References

Buma, L.E., Vluggen, S., Zwakhalen, S., Kempen, G.I., and Metzelthin, S. (2022) 'Effects on clients' daily functioning and common features of reablement interventions: a systematic literature review', *European Journal of Ageing*, 17(5): 416.

Legg, L., Gladman, J., Drummond, A., and Davidson, A. (2016) 'A systematic review of the evidence on home care reablement services', *Clinical Rehabilitation*, 30(8): 741–9.

Metzelthin, S., Rostgaard, T., Parsons, M., and Burton, E. (2020) 'Development of an internationally accepted definition of reablement: a Delphi study', *Ageing and Society*, 42(3): 703–18.

Thuesen, J., Feiring, M., Doh, D., and Westendorp, R. (2021) 'Reablement in need of theories of ageing: would theories of successful ageing do', *Ageing & Society*, 1–13. DOI: 10.1017/S0144686X21001203

Index

References to figures appear in *italic* type;
those in **bold** refer to tables.

A

active ageing 40, 42, 49
active and healthy ageing 246
  rhetorical frames of 59, 62, 241
  travelling of ideas of 46, 50, *60*
activities of daily living (ADL) 34, 95, 98,
  99, 108, 129, 221
  Barthel ADL Index 130
  functional independence in **126**, 129,
  131, 132
  Instrumental Activities of Daily Living
  (IADLs) 95, 99, 129, 130, 221
  instruments used to measure 131
  Nottingham Extended Activities of Daily
  Living (NEADL) 130
  Personal Activities of Daily Living
  (PADL) 129
  satisfaction of performance of **127**
  training 35
Adult Social Care Outcomes Toolkit
  (ASCOT) 102, 104, 106, **129**, 152
adverse events **124**, 127
ageing 222
  approach to ageing in Australia 54
  and healthy ageing 23
  International Federation of Ageing (IFA)
  Copenhagen Summit 49
  models of 223
  OECD active and productive ageing
  policy 49
  population 4–5
  successful 40
  WHO 2015 World Report on Ageing
  and Health 49
  see also active and healthy ageing
Alzheimer's disease 164
  see also dementia
assessment of need 7, 31
Assessment of Quality of Life (AQOL)
  scale 102
Australasia 21, 30, 41, 48
  characteristics of **22**
  development of reablement services
  in 53–5
Australia 10, 12, 21, 23, 41, 48, 62,
  81, 133
  aboriginal and Torres Strait islander
  people 30
  availability of health-related services to
  individuals with dementia 180

characteristics of **22**
client-level outcomes and measurement
  instruments **120–2**
Commonwealth Home Support
  Programme (CHSP) 54
COPE intervention 174
facilitation of reablement 83
funding model of reablement 30
implementation of reablement 84
Interdisciplinary Home-Based
  Reablement Program (I-HARP) 176
interventions for individuals with
  dementia in 179
LifeFul intervention **173**, 177
national forum for home and community
  services 54
national policy documents approach to
  ageing 54
National Primary Health Care Strategy 54
Personal Enablement Programme
  (PEP) 72
reablement in **24–9**
Regional Assessment Services (RAS) 72
restorative home care 53–4, 61
services delivered by reablement
  teams 31
Short-Term Restorative Care
  Programme 54
see also Western Australia
Austria 13
autonomous self-development 227
autonomy 228
autonomy-compatible reablement 219–37
  promotion of 229–31
  roles of the helper and doer 230

B

Bangor Goal Setting Interview (BGSI) 175
Barthel ADL Index 130
Bauer, A. 143, 154, 155
Befriending and Reablement Service
  (BARS) 99
Béland, D. 47, 50
Belgium 13
Beresford, B. 98, 102, 104, 105
bone fractures 9
boundary-blurring 8
boundary-making 8
Braun, V. and Clarke V., thematic analysis
  method 48

Buma, L. 36, 99, 244
Burton, E. 101

C

Canada 12, 103
Canadian Occupational Performance
  Measure (COPM) 34, 130, 175
Capacity for Development (Ellerman) 227
care needs, understanding and how to
  meet 195–6
care work
  implication of working with reablement
    for attractiveness of 201–7
  meaningfulness in 201, *202*
  and meeting client needs 201–4
  'responsibilisation' in 193
care workers 7–8, 16–17, 31, 247
  assessment of performance of 212
  cooperation with occupational therapists
    and physiotherapists 198
  experience of reablement for 15
  intentions to quit their job 207, *209*
  interpersonal skills in relationships with
    clients 193
  managerial support 199, 207, *208*
  meetings with managers/managerial
    attention 204–7
  prestige of reablement work for 199–200
  professional autonomy and
    flexibility 200–1
  providing individualised care 204, *205*
  providing reablement and finding
    meaningfulness in work 211
  reablement implementation and
    improvements in retention and
    recruitment of care workers 210
  reduction in long-term care 5
  relationship between clients and 196
  shortage of 213
  see also home care workers
Center for Epidemiological Studies
  Depression Scale (CESD) 104
CHEERS statement 142, 157
China 13
  population ageing in 4
Clare, Linda 166
client-level outcomes 93–117
  adverse events **127**
  confidence **127**
  daily functioning 95–9
  death **127**
  definition of 118
  functional independence in ADL **126**
  health-related quality of life **126**, 129
  and instruments in reablement 118–36
  most commonly examined 95
  physical functioning 99–102, **126**, 129
  psychological functioning **127**, 130
  quality of life 102–4

satisfaction of performance of ADL **127**
  sedentary behaviour 127
  types and measures of 109
clients 16
  motivation of 197–8, 210
  self-determination of 227
clinical controlled trials (CCTs) 99
clinicians, recommendations for 156
Clotworthy, A. 11, 16, 35, 131,
  240–1, 244
cluster randomised controlled trials,
  physical function 101
Cochrane, A. 98
Cochrane systematic review, quality of
  life 103
cognition 105
cognitive abilities 163
coherence, as a secondary outcome 106
Commonwealth Home Support
  Programme (CHSP) 54
comparative cluster analysis 119
compensatory strategies 6
confidence **127**
context, and reablement
  implementation 110
context construct 69, 81
  Denmark 75–6
  i-PAHRIS framework 75–8
  The Netherlands 76–7
  New Zealand 77
  Norway 77–8
  Western Australia 78
COOP/Wonka 102, 103
COPE (Care of Persons with dementia in
  their Environment) intervention 170–4
cost-benefit analysis 140
cost-effectiveness analysis 138–9, 141–57
costs 154, 247
  healthcare 152
  overheads 155
  of reablement versus traditional home
    care 10
  for salaries 155
  and time-limited reablement
    programmes 231
cost-utility analysis 139
cultural contexts 12, 245
Czarniawska, Barbara 47

D

daily functioning 15, 95–9, 108
death **127**
decision analytic modelling 141
decision-makers, recommendations
  for 156
Delphi, definition of reablement 8, 21, 32,
  131, 239–40
Delphi study 6, 221, 240
dementia 9, 15, 163–88, 247

approaches to supporting individuals with dementia and their family members 166
balancing restorative and compensatory measures 167
challenges of reablement in dementia care 179–80, 181
characteristics of 164
classification of stages of 164–5
common features across reablement intervention programs in dementia care 178–9
COPE (Care of Persons with dementia in their Environment) intervention 170–4
dementia-specific skills among health professionals 167
diagnosis delays and access to reablement programs 180
as a disability 166
dyadic focus 167
effective reablement intervention programs for individuals with 168, 169–79
experience of reablement for people with 15
focus on independence 167
incidence of 164
individuals with dementia as target group for reablement 33
interference with an individual's ability to do everyday activities 163–5
occupational therapists visits to 174
physical home environment improvements 168
psychosocial interventions 168
reablement in dementia care compared to standard reablement 166–7
reablement intervention programs for individuals with 171–3
suggested techniques for reablement in dementia care 168, 169
supporting the informal care partner 169
theories about dementia and opportunities for therapeutic efforts 165–6
Denmark 12, 13, 21, 41, 48, 55, 62, 133
Association of Occupational Therapists 72
characteristics of 22
client-level outcomes and measurement instruments 122
'Coffee first' homecare 231–2
context construct of reablement 75–6
Dan Age 79, 83
delivery of reablement 82
development of reablement services in 56–8
education and resourcing 81
education and training in reablement 211

everyday rehabilitation 57, 61
facilitation of reablement 78–9, 83
Fredericia 49, 50, 57, 61, 70, 78
funding of reablement 76
implementation of reablement 84
implications of introduction of reablement for home care workers in 15, 189–216
individuals with dementia as target group for reablement 180
innovation construct and delivery of reablement in 70
integration of reablement within home care 81
long-term care and reablement care work in 190–1
National Board of Social Services 79
National Health Board 76, 79
New Public Management (NPM) steering principles 191
proportion of older people receiving reablement 30
reablement in 24–9, 49, 50, 57, 70, 190
recipient construct of reablement 72–3
services delivered by reablement teams 31
social and healthcare assistants 191
Social Services Act (2014) 61
staff providing reablement services 83
training in reablement 31
depression/mood, as a secondary outcome 104
disability
incidence of 4
United Nations Convention on the Rights of Persons with Disabilities 166
disruptive innovation 226
Doh, D. 220, 221, 222, 225, 226, 229
Duke Social Support Index 105
Dutch EASYCare study 103

E

EADL (Extended Activities of Daily Living) 129
education
and resourcing 81
role in reaching client's goals 35
and training in reablement 211
Ellerman, David P. 227, 228
Empowerment Theory 40
Enablement Theory 40
England 21, 41, 62
assessment of need 31
Department of Health Care Services Efficiency Delivery Programme 51
development of reablement services in 51–2
funding model of reablement 30–1
goals of reablement 30

reablement in **24–9**
reablement training 31
services delivered by reablement teams 31
see also United Kingdom
environmental adaptations 35
ethnicity, of participants reablement
    studies 12
European Commission 49
European Quality of Life Scale
    (EQ-5D-5L) 102, 104, 130
European Union, policy on active
    ageing 49
EuroQoL thermometer visual analogue
    scale 104
everyday rehabilitation 30, 56, 61, 224
Evetts, J. 192, 193, 210
evidence, of the effectiveness of an
    intervention 94

F
facilitation context 69, 78–80, 83
    Denmark 78–9
    The Netherlands 79
    New Zealand 78
    Norway 78
    Western Australia 79–80
Fair Access to Care Services (FACS)
    Criteria 105
falls
    Falls Efficacy Scale 130
    increase in 105
    Modified Falls Efficacy Scale
        (MFES) 130
    prevention interventions 110
family members, support of 8, 166
Feiring, M. 12, 14, 21, 93, 101, 109, 241
Friedson, E. 192
functional disorder management 35
functional independence, in activities of
    daily living **126**, 129, 131, 132
functionality 221
function-focused care for the cognitively
    impaired (FFC-CI) **173**, 177–8
funding models 30–1, 76, 77, 245–6

G
gender, as factor regarding benefits from
    reablement 9
General Health Questionnaire
    (GHQ-12) 106
general rehabilitation 56
Gitlin, L. 174
Glendinning, C. 107, 154, 155
goals 225–6
    Bangor Goal Setting Interview
        (BGSI) 175
    goal-facilitation tool 231
    goal-oriented cognitive rehabilitation
        (GREAT trial) **171**, 175–6

goal-setting 40, 81–2, 225
    holistic approach to 34–5
    self-identified 225
goal-setting and goal-setting
    instruments 33–4
    Canadian Occupational Performance
        Measure (COPM) 34, 130, 175
    Towards Achieving Realistic Goals for
        Elders Tool (TARGET) instrument 34
Graff, L. 15, 36, 244
grand-level theory 242

H
health- and social care personnel 36
health economic evaluation of
    reablement 137–41, 155
    charting data and reporting results 143
    choice of health outcomes 152
    cost-benefit analysis 140
    cost-effectiveness and cost-utility
        analysis 138–40
    cost-effectiveness studies 153–4
    cost-minimisation and cost-analysis 138
    identification of focus points for 142
    published studies on **144–51**
    in relation to conventional home
        care 152
    study perspectives and estimated
        costs 152
    target groups 143
    time horizon 140–1, 152
Health of the Nation Outcome Scale
    (HONOS) 105
health professionals, perspectives of 239
health-related quality of life
    (HRQoL) 107, 129, 131–2
healthy and active ageing *see* active and
    healthy ageing
helping people help themselves 16, 227
Hjelle, K.M. 107
home care 16, 68–90, 212
    ageing-in-place 53
    assessment of an older person's needs 231
    in Denmark 190
home care assistance program **172**, 177
home care reablement services 59
home care workers
    in Denmark 191
    implications of introduction of
        reablement for 189–216
    see also care workers
Home Independence Program (HIP) 53,
    72, 79, 101
home rehabilitation 56, 61

I
Iceland 13
implementation-evaluation methods
    244

incremental cost-effectiveness ratios
(ICER) 157
independence 167, 221, 229
see also functional independence
innovation construct 68–9
  Denmark 70
  The Netherlands 70
  New Zealand 70–1
  Norway 71
  reablement within 80
  Western Australia 71–2
institutionalism 38
Instrumental Activities of Daily Living
  (IADLs) 95, 99, 129, 130, 221
instruments in reablement, client-level
  outcomes and 118–36
Interdisciplinary Home-Based Reablement
  Program (I-HARP) **172**, 176
interdisciplinary teams 36, 41, 62, 82, 193,
  210, 221
intermediate care 51, 52, 59
International Federation of Ageing (IFA)
  Copenhagen Summit 49
interpersonal skills, of care workers in
  relationships with clients 193
interpretivism 38
inter-RAI home care 74, 77, 81, 130
intervention costs 142, 154–5
intervention effects 156
interventions 41
  content of 244
  designed for individuals living with
    dementia 15
  intensive and relation-based 35–6
  multimodal 35
  person-centred 32–3
i-PAHRIS framework 68, 69, 72,
  75–8, 81
Ireland 12
Italy 12, 13
  home care assistance program 177
Iwarsson, S. 97, 100

J

Japan 13, 133
  client-level outcomes and measurement
    instruments 119, **122**, 133

K

Kitwood, Tom 166
Kjerstad, E. 153, 154

L

Langeland, E. 98, 101, 102
Law of Unintended Rewards 228
Legg, L. 37, 98, 109, 239
Lewin, G. 10, 15, 48, 53, 98, 102, 103,
  131, 153, 155, 219, 244
liberalism 38

LifeFul intervention **173**, 177
Lifestyle Exercise program (LiFe) 101
local bottom-up initiatives 30
long-term care (LTC) 11, 189
  bottom-up enabling approach to 63
  reduction in workers in 5
  shortage of care workers in 213
low-income countries 246

M

Mair, M. 106, 154, 156
Mansson, Marita 56
McLeod, B. 106, 154, 156
measurement instruments, for client-level
  outcomes **128–9**, 130
Medical Health Outcomes Study – mental
  health subscale 103
mental health
  General Health Questionnaire
    (GHQ-12) 106
  Medical Health Outcomes Study –
    mental health subscale 103
  Warwick Edinburgh Mental Health
    Wellbeing Scale (WEMWBS) 105
meta-range level theory 242
Metzelthin, S. 221, 239
micro-range level theory 242
mid-range level theory 242
minority ethnic groups, reablement and
  cultural values of 245
mobility 100
model-based studies 155
Modified Falls Efficacy Scale (MFES) 130
Moe, A. 107
mood, as secondary client-level
  outcome 104–5
Mood indicators – Minimum dataset 105
moral framework 11
motivation 197–8
  external 228
  intrinsic 228, 230
muscle memory 223

N

narrative emplotment 222
Nelson, Michelle 238
Netherlands, the 13, 21, 22, 41, 133
  Buurtzorg homecare provider 231–2
  characteristics of **22**
  client-level outcomes and measurement
    instruments **122**
  context construct of reablement 76–7
  Dutch Healthcare Authority 77
  facilitation construct of reablement 79
  funding models 31, 76, 77
  implementation of reablement 84
  occupational therapist/physiotherapist
    role in daily intervention 31
  reablement in **24–9**, 30, 70, 81

reablement training 31
recipient construct of reablement 73
'Stay Active at Home' programme 70,
    73, 77, 79
use of registered nurses to assess and
    coordinate services 82
use of the term 'reablement' in 30
New Zealand 12, 13, 21, 41, 48, 62, 129,
    133, 226
ageing-in-place initiatives 55
characteristics of 22
client-level outcomes and measurement
    instruments 122–4
Community FIRST restorative home
    care practice 55
context construct of reablement 77
District Health Boards (DHBs) 54
facilitation of reablement 79, 83
funding models 31, 77
health and social care 71
Health Strategy 55
Healthy Ageing Strategy 55
implementation of reablement 84
integration of reablement services within
    home care 81
inter-RAI home care and contact
    assessments 74
job satisfaction of care workers 200, 211
Māori population 30, 245
reablement in 24–9, 70–1
recipient construct of reablement 73–4
refinement of reablement service
    provision 81
restorative home support 54–5, 61
services delivered by reablement
    teams 31
Towards Achieving Realistic Goals for
    Elders Tool (TARGET) instrument 34
training for clinicians in using goal-
    setting tools 81
use of registered nurses to assess and
    coordinate services 82
Nordic care model 191
Nordic NORDCARE study 194
Northern Ireland 59, 62
development of reablement services
    in 52–3
Health and Social Care Trusts
    (HSCT) 52, 53
Norway 12, 21, 41, 48, 55, 62, 129,
    133, 211
characteristics of 22
client-level outcomes and measurement
    instruments 124
context construct of reablement 77–8
delivery of reablement in 82
development of reablement services
    in 58–9, 61
everyday rehabilitation 58, 61

facilitation of reablement 79, 83
factors that influence individual's success
    with reablement 107
funding models 30
implementation of reablement in 71, 84
Innovation in the Care Services
    Report 58
integration of rehabilitation and home
    care resources 81
job satisfaction of care workers in 200
Norwegian Ministry of Health and Care
    Services 77
occupational therapist/physiotherapist
    role in daily intervention 31
Occupational Therapy Association 58,
    71, 79, 83
reablement in 24–9, 30, 71
recipient construct of reablement 74–5
refinement of reablement service
    provision 81
services delivered by reablement
    teams 31
staff providing reablement services 83
training for clinicians in using goal-
    setting tools 81
Nottingham Extended Activities of Daily
    Living (NEADL) 130
nurses
    integration in the reablement
        interventions 73
    use to assess and coordinate services 82
    visits to individuals with dementia 174

O

occupational professionalism 193
occupational therapists 13, 31, 36, 174
OECD, active and productive ageing
    policy 49
older person/people 16
    assessment of needs during
        homecare 231
    improving physical functionality of 16
organisational issues 211
organisational professionalism 193
organisations, providing reablement
    services 83
outcomes
    'if this, then that' 223
    see also client-level outcomes

P

pain 105
paradigmatic cases 194
Parsons, John 14, 16, 32, 47, 93, 101,
    109, 238
Parsons, M. 98
Personal Activities of Daily Living
    (PADL) 129
Pettersson, C. 97, 100

Philadelphia Geriatric Centre Morale Scale
(PGCMS) 105
philosophy, of reablement 220
Physical Activity Scale for the Elderly
(PASE) 101
physical and/or functional exercises 35
physical function 16, 99–102, **126**, 129,
131, 132, 223, 247
evidence for the effect of reablement
on 108
mobility 100
Short Form 36 (SF36) Health
Survey 100, 102, 103, 130
Short Physical Performance Battery
(SPPB) 99, 101, 130
physical rehabilitation 222
physiotherapists 31, 36
policy makers 110
political agenda-setting 47, 50
population ageing 4–5
positivism 38
post-positivism 38
PROFANE (Prevention of Falls Network
Europe) 110
professionalism 192
psychological functioning **127**, 130,
131, 132

Q

quality of life 102–4, 107
Assessment of Quality of Life (AQOL)
scale 102
health-related **126**, 131–2
quality-adjusted life-years
(QALYs) 139, 140

R

Rahja, M. 9, 15, 157, 240
randomised controlled trials (RCTs) 94,
98, 99, 141
ReAble Network 6, 13, 16, 48, 110, 143,
238, 239, 244
reablement
aim of 220
application and implementation of 13
approach to home care for
older people 3
appropriateness of 31
central goal of 221
as a cost-effective option 137–60
current situation 219–20
definition of 5, 6–7, 8, 21, 32, 56, 109,
131, 239–40, 244
effect on outcomes 9–11
effectiveness of 11
experience of 15
and facilitating change 196–7
features of 80–1, 220–1
focus of 240–2

goal of 225
grand theory level 38
health-economic perspectives on 15
impact on perceptions and experiences of
staff 244
implementation of 68, 84, 242–3, 246
implications of 11–12
and the introduction of new tasks and
methods 197–8
lessons learnt about 245–6
liminal nature of 241
long-term effects of 244
origin and features of 224–7
as policy and practice 12
prestige of reablement work 199–200
problems of 222–4
publications on 13, 224
purpose of 239–40
relation to rehabilitation 5–6
research on 12–13, 220–1, 244
spread of 12–13, 84
studies of 108, 211
task-shifting practices in 8
theoretical aspects of 37–41, 42, 242
travelling of ideas of 47, 48–50, 59,
219, 242
reablement models 23–31, 109, 240
in familiar settings 33
features of 31–7, 41
goal-setting and goal-setting
instruments 33–4
holistic approach to goals 34–5
intensive and relation-based
interventions 35–6
interdisciplinary teams 36
multimodal intervention components 35
national guidance 30
person-centred interventions 32–3
policy/program goals 30
regular assessments of individual's
functional capacities 37
staff training 37
targeted at home-dwelling older
adults 33
transferring between countries/
jurisdictions 85
reablement services
involvement of users in measuring impact
of 110
outcome measures 105–6
reablement teams 31
reablement theory
governmentality perspective 40
grand theory level **39**, 42
meta-range level **39**, 40, 42
micro-range level **39**, 40, 42
mid-range level **39**, 40
recipient construct 69, 72–5, 81
Denmark 72–3

The Netherlands 73
New Zealand 73–4
Norway 74–5
Western Australia 75
rehabilitation
everyday rehabilitation 30, 56, 61, 224
physical 222
relation of reablement to 5–6
research
impact of services within 15
on reablement 98, 243–5
researchers, recommendations for 156–7
residential aged care homes 181
reablement intervention programs for
individuals with dementia in 178
restorative home care/home support/
care 17, 30
retrospective study designs 155
rhetorical frames 47
Rostgaard, T. 15, 36, 167, 238, 244
Rowe, J.W. 40
Ryburn, B. 107

S

Scandinavia 10, 22, 41, 61, 154, 241
characteristics of **22**
development of reablement services
in 55–9
everyday rehabilitation 30, 224
long-term care policy 56
providers of reablement 31
see also Denmark; Norway; Sweden
Scotland 59, 62
development of reablement services
in 52
evaluation of reablement services in 106
sedentary behaviour 127
self-assessment, STAR tool 106
self-reports
daily functioning 95
physical functioning 100–1
Sense of Coherence questionnaire
(SOC-13) 106
Senior, H.E. 104
Sense of Coherence questionnaire
(SOC-13) 106
service evaluations 104, 105
service providers 110
Short Form 36 (SF36) Health Survey 100,
102, 103, 108, 130
Short Physical Performance Battery
(SPPB) 99, 101, 130
Silver Chain 53, 72, 79, 83
Sims-Gould, J. 94, 97, 100, 102, 103, 105
Slater, P. 99
social connectivity 222, 247
social functioning 132
social scientists, perspectives of 239
social support 105

South Korea 13
staff training 37, 82–3
STAR tool 106
'Stay Active at Home' programme 70, 73,
77, 79
study designs, retrospective 155
support workers see care workers
Sweden 12, 13, 21, 41, 48, 55, 62, 133
caring skills of health professionals in
home care for older people 230
characteristics of **22**
client-level outcomes and measurement
instruments **124–5**
development of reablement services
in 61
everyday rehabilitation 56, 224
population 65 years or older 23
reablement in **24–9**, 30
services delivered by reablement
teams 31
Swedish Association of Occupational
Therapists, definition of reablement 56
systematic reviews 95, **96**, 243

T

Taiwan 12, 129, 133
client-level outcomes and measurement
instruments **125**
target groups 8–9
teamwork 82
Tessier, A. 97, 100, 103
therapists, cooperation with 198–9
Thuesen, J. 9, 15, 38, 157, 240, 241
time horizons, retrospective study
designs 155
Timed Up and Go (TUG) test 99,
100, 130
Tinetti, M.E. 100, 224
Towards Achieving Realistic Goals for
Elders Tool (TARGET) instrument 34
training 31, 37, 82–3
for clinicians in using goal-setting
tools 81
in reablement 31, 211
treatment plans, adherence to 225
Treatment Theory 40
trial designs 141
model-based 141
randomised controlled trials (RCTs) 141
Tuntland, H. 10, 14, 15, 70, 94, 95, 98,
102, 103, 109, 238, 242
Canadian Occupational Performance
Measure (COPM) 175
client-level outcomes 93
cost-effectiveness studies 153, 154
goals of clients 34

U

'unhelpful help' 220, 228, 229

United Kingdom 10, 12, 13, 48, 130, 133
  Befriending and Reablement Service
    (BARS) 99
  characteristics of **22**
  client-level outcomes and measurement
    instruments **125**
  development of reablement in 50–3
  goal-oriented cognitive rehabilitation
    (GREAT trial) 175–6
  reablement in Essex County 110–11
  service evaluation 106
  see also England
United Nations Convention on the Rights
    of Persons with Disabilities 166
United Nations Development Programme
    (UNDP) 227
United States 12
  COPE intervention 170–4
  function-focused care for the cognitively
    impaired (FFC-CI) 177–8

V

Vik, K. 211

W

Wales 62
  development of reablement services
    in 52
  travel of reablement to 59
walking impairment scale 100
Warwick Edinburgh Mental Health
    Wellbeing Scale (WEMWBS) 105
welfare regimes 22

Westendorp, R. 11, 16, 35, 131, 238,
    240–1, 244
Western Australia
  Aged Care Policy Directorate 80
  Commonwealth Home Support
    Programme (CHSP) 78
  context construct of reablement 78
  delivery of reablement 82–3
  facilitation construct of
    reablement 79–80
  Home Independence Programme
    (HIP) 53, 72, 79, 80, 101
  innovation construct of reablement
    71–2
  recipient construct of reablement 75
  WA State Government Home and
    Community Care Programme (WA
    HACC) 72, 80
  see also Australia
Whitehead, P.J. 95, 97, 99, 103, 104,
    105, 107
Wilde, A. 107
Winkel, A. 98
World Health Organization (WHO)
  2015 World Report on Ageing and
    Health 49
  definition of compensatory strategies 6
  definition of rehabilitation 5
  and dementia as a public health
    priority 164

Z

Zingmark, M. 10, 15, 143, 154, 155, 156

Printed and bound by CPI Group (UK) Ltd, Croydon, CR0 4YY

27/10/2024

14580560-0003